REVEALING
GRACE

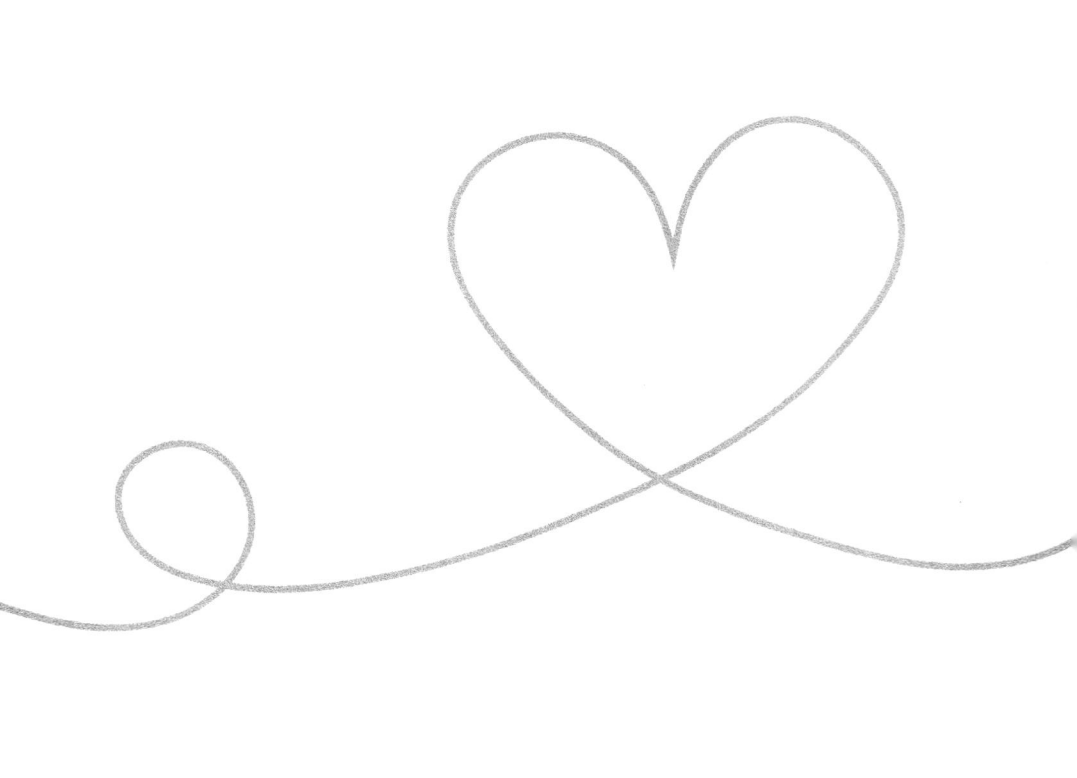

REVEALING
GRACE

A STORY ABOUT A CANCER ADVENTURE
AND A COMMUNITY

AMY CONN

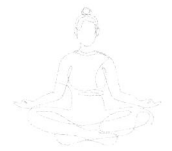

YOGA FOR WELLNESS

Revealing Grace – A Story About a Cancer Adventure and a Community
Copyright © 2025 by Amy Conn

All rights reserved, including the right to reproduce distribute, or transmit in any form or by any means. Except as permitted under the U.S. Copyright Act of 1976, no part of this book may be reproduced, distributed, or transmitted in any form or by any means, or stored in a database or retrieval system without the written permission of the authors, except in the case of brief passages embodied in critical reviews and articles where the title, author and ISBN accompany such review or article.

For information contact:
amyconnyoga@gmail.com

amyconnyoga.com

Published by:
Yoga for Wellness

Cover design by SantoRoy71

Interior book design by Francine Platt, Eden Graphics, Inc.

Paperback ISBN 979-8-89454-015-3

eBook ISBN 979-8-89454-016-0

Library of Congress Control Number: 2024915720

Manufactured in the United States of America

First Edition

*Dedicated to Michael,
who pays attention to the details of my heart;
and to Benjamin and Abigail, who hold it.*

A portion of proceeds from the sale of this book will be donated to **Survivor Wellness** —a nonprofit organization. Survivor Wellness is dedicated to supporting the cancer survivor community.

Table of Contents

FOREWORD IX

── **PART ONE – ME** ──

"You Have Breast Cancer" 3
Walking into My New World 11
Telling People 25
The Bald Party 33
Conversations on a Mountain Peak 39
Five Bottles 43
Lists on a Whiteboard 47
White Noise 51
The Vice Patrol 53
Kickback 57
Eyelashes 59

── **PART TWO – MY FAMILY** ──

Meeting Michael 65
Benjamin's Window 71
Abigail's Swing 77
Mashed Potato Day 81

── **PART THREE – MY COMMUNITY** ──

Firefighters 85
Tarot Reading 91
Rose 95
My "Y" 99
Moving Past the Fear 103
So Now What? 105

REMEMBERING, MEMORIALIZING	109
BEYOND THE SHADOW OF DOUBT	115
AMAZING STORIES	119
THE WORK BEHIND THE WORK	121
COUNTING TAXIS	123
C IS FOR "COMMUNITY"	133
COFFEE, TEA, AND COMMUNITY	137
GIRLFRIENDS FOREVER	141
AT THE OYSTER BAR WITH THE BREAST CANCER GIRLS	145
CASTING PARTY	149
WALKING ANGELS	153
THE NUMBERS GAME	159
BEING "PRO-ACTIVE"	165
BEING CAPABLE	171
NOTICING SUNSETS AGAIN	173
FUND-RAISING	179
HOLDING OPEN THE SPACE	185
LETTING GO OF PAIN	187

PART FOUR – MY WORLD

MY DREAM OF YOGA	193
WOMEN BEYOND CANCER	197
SUNDANCE YOGA RETREAT	207
REPRIEVE	215
TERRILYN	219
BLESSING	225
ABOUT THE AUTHOR	227
ACKNOWLEDGMENTS	228

"If you pay attention at every moment, you form a new relationship to time. In some magical way, by slowing down, you become more efficient, productive, and energetic, focusing without distraction directly on the task in front of you. Not only do you become immersed in the moment, you become that moment."

– MICHAEL RAY, *The Highest Goal*

Foreword

by Charlotte Bell

It would be difficult to find a person—any person—whose life hasn't been affected by cancer in some way. According to statistics from the National Cancer Institute, 41 percent of all men and women will be diagnosed with some form of cancer in their lifetimes. Some of these cancers will be mild and easily treated; others will require aggressive treatment. Some people will bounce back after treatment and never again experience cancer. Others will bounce back only to face cancer again. For others, cancer will take over their bodies, leaving them only the choice to vacate.

But cancer is not just a set of statistics; it has a face. That face is bigger than we might think at first glance. The face of cancer is the face of the person in the process of living with cancer. It is the face of that person's spouse and children, friends and family. It is the face of the health professionals and wellness practitioners that guide us through the process and soften the sharp edges. It is the face of the community of cancer survivors that a person meets during the journey, the people who can truly understand the physical, mental, emotional and spiritual implications of living with cancer. Finally, it is the face of those who generously, unexpectedly appear to lend support—some we already knew and others that the cancer experience has gifted us.

This is what Amy's book has taught me. While much of the cancer journey is a trail the survivor walks alone, its reach is as wide as the sky. It delves deep into the subterranean levels of our beings while simultaneously touching everyone we encounter. It is both difficult and enlightening. It strengthens our bonds with the beings around us—human and animal. It teaches us to recognize the preciousness of this day, this moment.

This book is not only a how-to book on living gracefully with cancer, although it certainly offers wise counsel and practical suggestions. It is also a companion, a gentle guide to light the terrain ahead. It is a friend that will not lie to you about the sometimes crushing challenges our bodies, hearts and minds will face. Most of all, it speaks from the voice of a yogi, a voice that gets bogged down in the day-to-day difficulties of living with cancer only temporarily, because as a yogi, Amy knows that the minutiae of living with cancer is always only a small part of a much bigger picture.

So many of my friends and family members, including Amy, have made the cancer journey and come out the other side a different person—more present, more appreciative, more grateful for the gift of this day. My wish for those whose hands this lovely book happens to find is that they read it slowly, savor it, reflect on their own experience, and look for the bigger picture that Amy has so gracefully brought to life."

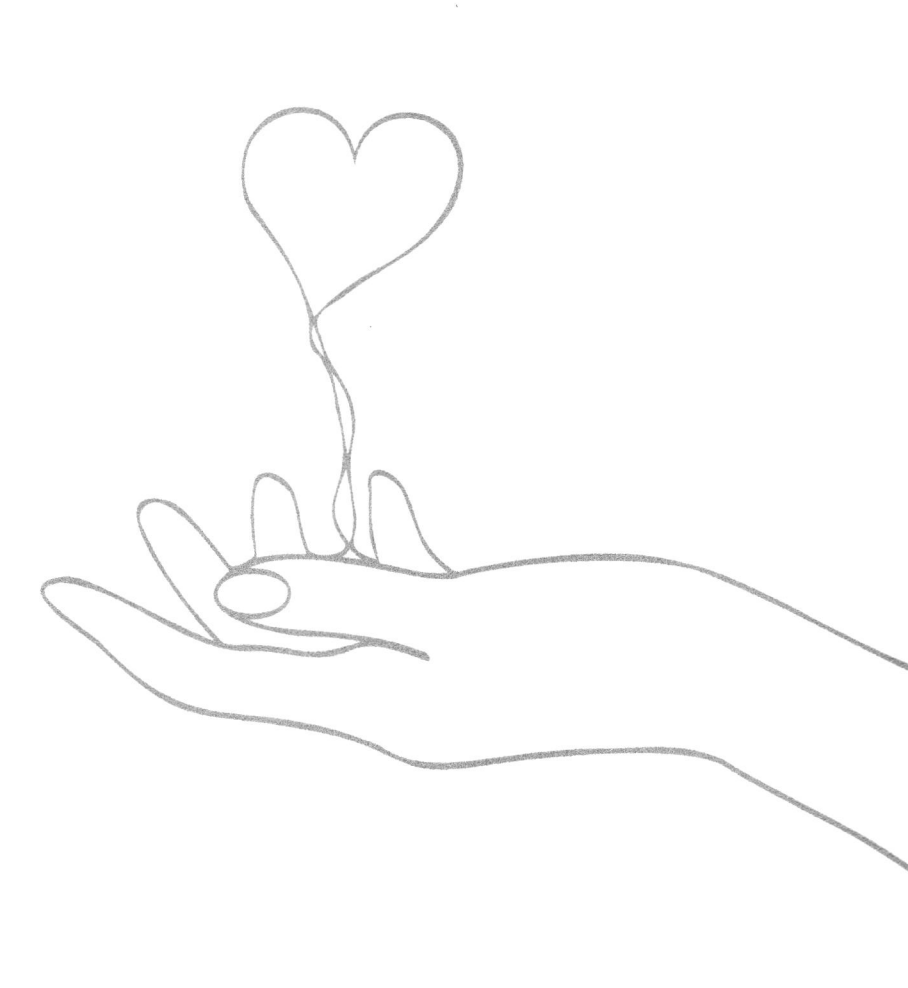

PART ONE *Me*

"The secret of cancer is to not feed it, not give it any recognition beyond what is necessary, not give it attention. Rather, love the working, healthy parts of the body. Love the parts that are nourishing and life-giving. Self-acceptance begins with the self."

– AMY CONN

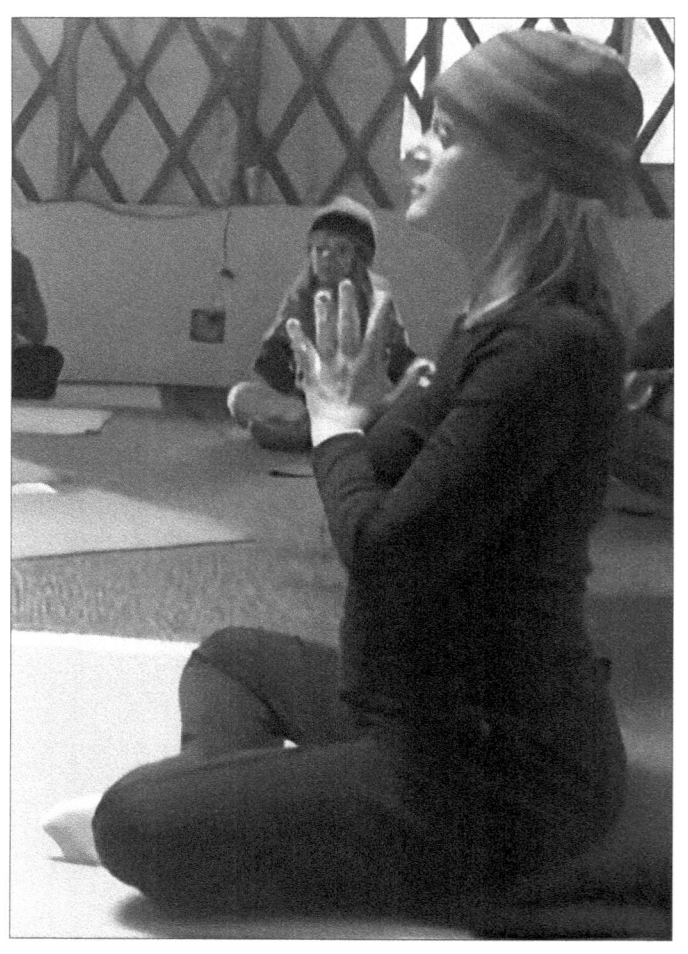

"You Have Breast Cancer"

There are sounds to seasons. There are sounds to places, and there are sounds to every time in one's life.

—Alison Wyrley Birch

On Abigail's fifth birthday, we decided to take her entire preschool class ice skating.

I remember asking Michael, "What were we thinking? Preschoolers can barely stand without falling down."

We were ice skating at the rink with a dozen of our daughter's classmates; *all* of us concentrating heavily on staying injury-free. When my cell phone rang, I half expected it to be a concerned parent worried that their child might have sliced their finger with the blade of a skate.

Instead, the voice on the other end told me to come in for a biopsy. I remember circling around the rink, putting my cell phone back in my pocket, and looking over at Michael, holding up three skidding four and five-year-olds.

I skated up behind him. "We have an appointment."

He looked at me for a brief, yet suspended, moment before speaking. Then, without any hesitation in his voice he said, "Okay."

I skated on, scooping up two more kids. And there we had it. The ball was in play, right in the middle of our life.

The spring thaw began early that year. I was a little over a month out from running the Salt Lake City Marathon. Sitting in a dark examining room with only the illumination from the ultrasound machine, and perhaps the small stream of light sneaking in from underneath the door separated me from the rest of the office.

My radiologist, Dr. Clark, was concerned about a lump he saw. The ultrasound confirmed the next step, a biopsy. He told me he'd be forwarding his findings to Dr. Blumenthal, my newly appointed surgeon, and to Dr. Cannon, my friend and OB GYN.

What he said next surprised me, but I was grateful for it just the same. "I'll have the results this evening. Here is my home phone number. You're welcome to call me tonight."

I took the card as he motioned to the door. "Now go one door down. My assistant will make the appointments for you."

Still holding his card, I walked numbly to the next door as instructed.

Dr. Clark is an enthusiastic physician, and we had chatted a lot during my appointments about my up-coming marathon and his own love for sports and the outdoors.

"I have four active children who keep me on the move all the time," he joked, but I could tell he was in shape. And he didn't seem to think that talking about his four children would somehow contaminate his professional image. Instead, that touch of vulnerability assured me that he was probably honest in other areas of his life as well.

People often say, "My kids keep me on the go all the time." But that usually means that they're endlessly playing taxi for them. This man actually played with his kids, ran with and skied with them. His integrity appealed to me, and I found myself listening to the sound of its underlying meaning.

I walked into the next room and sat down. I could feel my world changing. The room was carefully decorated to communicate peace—a good thing, considering the nightmares that brought most people here.

Muted lighting, soft music, and a comfy chair. The assistant had a soft voice—I'm sure Dr. Clark told me her name, but I couldn't remember it. She sat within arm's reach, but when she spoke, it seemed she was miles away.

She continued making appointments for me. Somehow, I was able to follow along without cross-checking calendars. It shouldn't have been possible for the list of appointments to fit into my family's hectic schedule.

"Good," she seemed satisfied with her find. "I have an appointment available for you tomorrow morning with Dr. Blumenthal. She is a referral of Dr. Cynthia Cannon." She looked up from her computer. "Will that work for you?"

I nodded as my mind drifted to my childhood friend.

Cindy Cannon is my OB-GYN. She delivered Abigail and had only been absent for two days during my whole pregnancy with Benjamin. Scorpio that my son is, always wanting to take matters into his own hands, Benjamin arrived on one of those two days. When Dr. Cannon delivered Abigail, she was five months pregnant with her own daughter. Now our children are in Girl Scouts together.

Cindy, and I grew up in the same Long Beach, California neighborhood. Cindy's brother knew my brother, Chris. Her father was a physician too and was always so very kind.

That's how my parents always described him. "He is a very kind man."

Cindy played the trumpet alongside my brother, Chris, in the Woodrow Wilson High School Jazz Band in 1980 when they won second place in the Monterey Jazz Festival. I remember coming home after school to find the entire band practicing in my parent's oversized bedroom where, according to my brother Chris the acoustics were just right.

I sometimes think of the irony of Cindy and I being together again, seven hundred miles east from where we first began.

The assistant handed me a piece of paper with the dates of my appointments. I still couldn't remember her name, and her hair covered her badge. Still numb, I walked out of the hospital.

I remember thinking I should put them away in my pocket, or in my purse. Instead, I held them in my hand as though they were tardy slips from the school secretary that I have to show to my homeroom teacher, then wait while she makes the proper marks in her attendance book.

I carried the slips across the street to the parking garage marked overhead, "For patients only."

I got into my car, but I just sat there. I didn't turn on the radio, I was only aware of the silence. I'm not sure for how long, but I knew Michael was waiting for me to call.

I looked in the rear-view mirror. The image looking back seemed unfamiliar.

Then, suddenly, everything fell into place.

My life is about to change, but I'm still me.

It was just two nights earlier when Michael had found the lump in my right breast. "Honey, you need to check this out."

I could hear worry in his voice, and I replaced his hand with mine to feel what he was feeling.

"Yes—okay." I had paused between the two responses.

I even surprised myself with my renunciative tone. I did not deny the lump nor argue his request. "I'll make the appointment to see the radiologist."

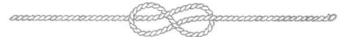

Dr. Regina Blumenthal shares her office with another surgeon. Michael held my hand while we waited.

Dr. Blumenthal is a slender woman and was once an aspiring ballerina.

Today she was running a little late. We'd brought Abigail, and she'd fallen asleep on her back across Michael's lap. He gently rubbed her belly.

I sat cross-legged in a chair adjacent to his. We didn't want to wake Abigail, so we didn't move except to turn our faces toward Dr. Blumenthal when she sat down across from me.

"How much do you know?" she asked.

"I chose not to call Dr. Clark. I wanted to get a good night's sleep."

She appeared relieved and bothered at the same time. "Ahhh, well. . ."

She held my file in her hand and half-gestured with it.

Is she going to open it?

"I'm glad you didn't call and I'm glad you got your rest. . ." Her voice trailed off again. She looked as if she wants to get up and pace the room, but she looked right at me. "You have breast cancer."

I know she kept talking, but I couldn't understand the words.

Michael reached out, with his other hand and didn't change his rhythm with Abigail, but I was out of reach except for the bottom of my shoe.

I could hear the sound of Michael rubbing the bottom of my shoe.

I was looking right at Dr. Blumenthal. I felt like I was alert, and attentive, but her words failed to penetrate my brain. All of my awareness was focused on those things connected to my heart.

I heard every breath Abigail took, saw every motion of Michael's hand as he continued to rub her tummy. All the while Dr. Blumenthal was explaining what she knows and what she doesn't know, her voice calm, warm, and yet, very far away.

Eventually a single tear escaped from my right eye. It slid

down my cheek, and I was surprised when the salt seeped into my mouth.

Suddenly I was fully present. The tear brought me back from my husband's touch, my daughter's breath, to my surgeon's voice and the new future she was spelling out.

"I have breast cancer." I was calm. This was not a question.

"Yes."

"Okay."

It occurred to me why she was late, because I'm about to make her late for her next patient. She seemed unconcerned, willing to sit with me while Michael and I digest this news and our next steps.

More talking, more explanation, and a sketchy map of the months ahead.

Dr. Blumenthal's assistant gives me more slips of paper, more appointments, and more tests. The predictable heaviness weighs on each of us as we walk out of the office, down the stairs, out of the building, and into the parking lot.

Abigail was walking and holding Michael's hand. She set the pace; there was no rush to make our next move.

This parking lot is different than the one outside the radiology building. The sun shines on our faces and warms the inside of the car. There was snow on the ground, but spring was approaching, and I could feel the change of the season around me. I was changing—so was my world.

Abigail climbed up into her car seat in the back and buckled up.

Michael checked her belt, shut her door, and then slid behind the wheel and looked at me.

He didn't seem to be breathing.

"I need to laugh tonight, Michael. Let's get a babysitter and see a funny movie or something. I need to feel lighter than I do right now."

He nodded.

My whole family has listened to Garrison Keillor's *Prairie*

Home Companion on NPR since we were young. I remember listening to it with my parents when we lived in California. My mother loved the stories and the character actors.

Our son, Benjamin, at eight, was a natural sound-effects guy; he could make car noises before he could walk. I have no explanation for this talent except that all of Michael's extended family is from the Detroit area and they're all immersed in the auto industry in one form or another. I call it the *Detroit gene.*

Fred Newman, the sound effects guy from *Prairie Home Companion*, was in town that very evening promoting his book, *Mouth Sounds*. It was being held at the art studio owned by a parent of one of my students at school, also a breast cancer survivor.

That night, Michael and I were part of the crowd squeezed into the studio listening to Fred Newman make elephant sounds, bird calls, the most amazing rendition of various baby cries, and the ever popular and quite familiar car sounds. I laughed until tears were running down my cheeks.

He brought me out of deterioration and into healing.

In a new strange and harsh world, he was familiarity—not that of my childhood but of the emotion and sound of my own laughter.

The vibration of my chest when I laughed out loud was a distinct reminder that I am more familiar with the person who laughs than with the person who mourns. This is not to say that one is more or less important than the other. Each has a purpose in our lives. Each is significant to living.

What I discovered through Fred Newman's virtuoso *mouth sounds* performance that evening was a rediscovery of Benjamin's *mouth sounds*, created, contained, and corrected. I needn't look farther than my own household to find the laughter that would heal my wounds.

As Dorothy in *The Wizard of Oz* said, "There's no place like home."

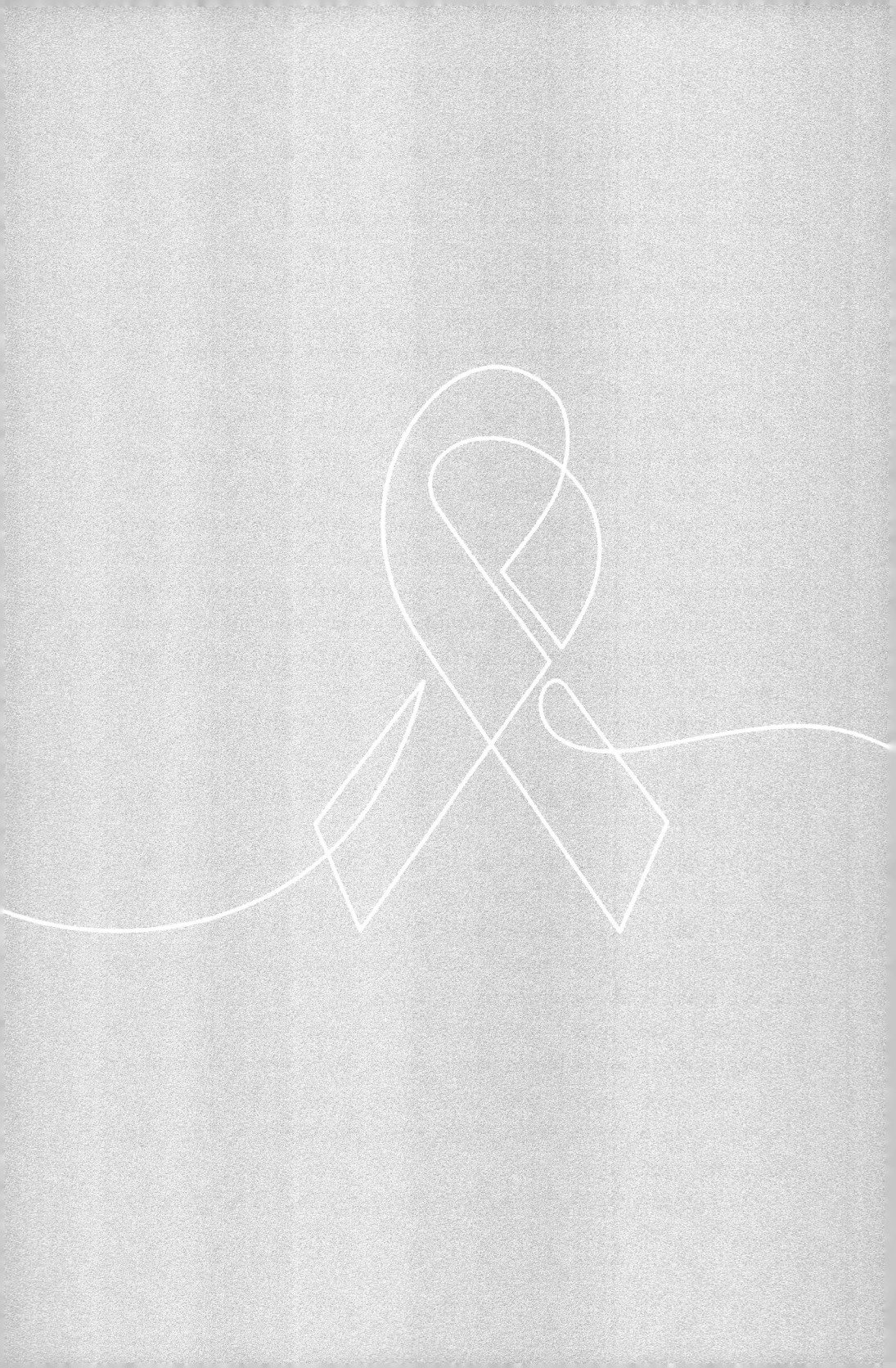

Walking into My New World

*It may be that when we no longer know what to do,
we have come to our real work, and when we no longer
know which way to go, we have begun our real journey.*

—Wendell Berry

When my breast cancer was diagnosed, I was practicing yoga four or five times a week. I contacted the owner of the studio and asked her what steps she recommended prior to my treatment and self-healing. I received only a moment of sadness before receiving her prescription for two things; restorative classes and—let's face it, daily doses of high cacao dark chocolate.

I was grateful for her response.

Ironically, I was in the tapering-down phase of a marathon training program. I had spent the past five months training for a race that was to take place in exactly one month. With the tremendous focus it had required, I wasn't ready to just leave it and leap over to the *let's train for cancer* track.

When we met with Dr. Blumenthal again. I asked about the propriety of continuing training if the required surgery was to be a lumpectomy. I looked straight into her eyes and heard myself say, "I understand about this surgery thing, but I'm running a marathon in a month. Do you have any problems with that?"

Dr. Blumenthal did a double-take, cocked her head to one side, glanced at Michael—apparently checking to see if he'd heard the same thing—and then quickly looked back at me—as though I hadn't noticed.

She responded in full surgeon mode. "I meet with a committee every Thursday morning. I will get back to you on this subject."

You see, until this point in time, I was the type of person who enjoyed predictability. In fact, I insisted upon it. I liked to know what to expect; I hated being blind-sided. I wanted to be prepared and if I had to change plans at the last minute, at least I would be changing an existing plan, not trying to come up with a brand new one from scratch.

When Michael and I started planning our family, I assumed that we could sail into parenthood in the same way I conceived my lesson plans, which I always had prepared nine or ten months in advance. My body had its own plan. When the months started slipping by with no pregnancy in sight, we made an appointment to talk about infertility with my OB-GYN.

Michael patiently explained to Dr. Cannon, "You gotta understand where she's coming from. She's the type of person who wants to conceive on a Monday, do the pregnancy that same week, and deliver on Friday, so that it doesn't conflict with the weekend."

Our two children are evidence that our fertility was not in question.

In my mind, my work with Dr. Blumenthal was no different. Can I fit cancer into the *big picture?*

When I got out of the meeting with Dr. Blumenthal, I called Paige Beals, my running partner. "Paige, you know how this marathon raises funds for the Huntsman Cancer Institute?"

"Sure."

I quickly continued. "Well, we have another, more personal, reason for running in April."

"What?"

I had to stop and swallow. I wasn't just making an announcement or a suggestion. I had a mission, and I desperately needed her to promote this mission with me. I needed her to believe in me as much as I believed in me. I knew I was going to be leaning on her psychologically.

"What?" she asked a second time.

"I just got diagnosed with breast cancer." I waited, letting every syllable sink in before I gave her any further details.

"What should we do?"

My heart melted at her use of, "We."

There was only one answer. I knew this instinctively, and once again I was faced with stating my request aloud. "I need us to continue training." I took a long breath and waited for her response.

"Okay." She paused. "Okay," she repeated, as if trying to convince herself.

Paige had been by my side for the past six months. We had trained through two seasons, shared countless stories of family drama, hardship, and celebration.

"Should I convince Amy to stop and refocus her diagnosis plan?" Might have been a question that passed through her mind. Instead, her words expressed simple support. "We can keep training."

And so, we did.

Next, I called my friend and trainer, Dawn Brockett. I had met her at the yoga studio also. An instructor and personal trainer, she understood the magic behind combining food and exercise better than anyone I had ever met or any book I had read. She can individualize an exacting calorie intake required to supply sufficient energy to finish a marathon. Watching Dawn calculate body mass with energy input and output is absolutely fascinating, and I trusted her knowledge of yoga and the mind-body connection. She knew I wasn't a fast runner, but I had endurance.

When I heard her voice, I gave to her what I was coming to think of as my Outing Speech. "I want to update you on my training, but I also need to inform you of a glitch."

"Yes?"

"I have breast cancer. I need you to help me design a graduated running schedule that will include a surgery in the middle of it."

Like Paige, a long moment of silence followed. Then, in full support, she focused on my request. Like Paige, she had just joined *Team Amy*. I desperately needed them both to be aligned with me toward a mutual goal, to finish this race.

They had been there for me—moment by moment, month by month.

I hung up feeling lighter, brighter. Paige and Dawn would simply continue to do what they had been doing all along, training with me. Breast cancer was just another element in the game-plan, adding focus, propelling us forward with compelling determination.

Running the marathon became my perfect metaphor for dealing with the cancer. Yes, it's sentiment, trite, a cliché. I would have rolled my eyes at it in a novel. Life, I learned, was not embarrassed by the trite.

Michael didn't waste any time rolling his eyes or second-guessing. When he sent out periodic newsletters updates to friends and family, he fell right into the rhythm. "Amy is now in her 10th mile of chemo-treatments. . ."

I read the journal of another runner being treated for Hodgkin's lymphoma while training for his race. He documented his journey using the metaphor of mile markers for his transfusion sessions. On some days he would feel so sick that he couldn't eat but not sick enough that he couldn't run. On the road, his friends would help him keep him at his desired pace. In the hospital, the nurses would help him keep his desired frame of mind. Running kept his thoughts focused forward; his action channeled into forward motion.

Reading his diary helped me run my own race, both cancer and marathon. He won a trophy for running the fastest in his age category, a feat that surprised even him. In the end, he survived his cancer and gave the trophy to his transfusion nurses who, in many ways, were running alongside him the entire time.

Michael and I had wanted to keep everything *normal* for the children until we had more information about what we were dealing with and exactly what we could tell them to expect. We told our friends, the Nuttings, who would pick up Benjamin and Abigail after school, the guy Michael had swapped shifts with, Paige, Dawn and my yoga instructors. Outside of this small circle of friends, we chose to wait until we had a *Cancer Plan*.

Our families were all out of state, so we had decided not to tell them until we knew more.

It sounds very self-centered; and in a way, that's exactly what it was. We turned inward, to find our centers, our core selves. Call it instinct, intuition, or privacy.

Before we could share something that scared us at a core level, Michael and I knew we needed to build that strength within, and between ourselves first.

I was still bolting up in the middle of the night with fears of leaving my children. I told Michael, "That's why I've been scrapbooking all these years, so they would remember me!"

Slowly regaining my breath, I knew I had to set aside the fear. He would rub my back until I could lay down in bed again. Then I would dream. The dreams were not filled with fear and my nights slowly became restful and uninterrupted. When I finally reached that point, we knew we were ready to begin sharing our news with more people.

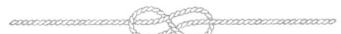

The morning of the surgery, we had to be at the hospital early, by 6:00 AM. We had the responsibility of the morning carpool for the children, and I insisted that Michael drive. I felt strongly about keeping to the morning routine. I didn't want the children's day in school to be haunted by terrible and scary thoughts. I wanted their environment to change as slowly as possible, giving them time to accept, adjust, and cope.

We had to wake Benjamin and Abigail early, around 5:30 AM, and keep them in their jammies, adding just a robe and slippers. Our routine often included juggling parent and kid schedules. As we bundled them into the car, we simply told the kids that Mommy had a doctor appointment and Daddy needed to drop me off. I'm sure it appears backwards to most people, but it felt right to us.

My family is my pod, and I wanted us together. I knew that, when I entered the hospital, I would be taking their courage, strength, and love with me. There was no fear, just movement through the routine.

At the hospital, I kissed both children and repeated my morning mantra, "Listen to your teachers."

They knew the Nuttings were going to be picking them up after school for a play date and they were very excited.

I kissed Michael and told him that I would be seeing him soon. Then I stepped out of the car and walked into my new world. One that I had not planned and had not expected. My family was my link between the world that I had helped create and the one that I was now creating, and I needed them with me this particular morning to help me make this transition.

Michael drove off with Benjamin and Abigail to begin the morning routine of preparing for school, brushing hair and teeth, eating breakfast, and packing lunches. He would get them ready, pick up the rest of the carpool, and drive them to school.

"Listen to your teachers!" he would remind them once again.

More kisses and hugs.

Then it would be time for Michael to begin the transition to our new world as he drove to the hospital and walked through the doors.

Both of my children were born at LDS Hospital in Salt Lake City, Utah. It's a place that holds magic for me. Michael and I took two courses to prepare for each child's birth, which were even filmed for a news program about non-medicated deliveries.

I had wonderful memories in the recovery rooms, celebrating their new lives with family and friends. I felt determined to keep the positive energy that I had held for this place.

The 6:00 AM crowd in the hospital's pre-surgical waiting room was not exuding magic. Clearly, no one had their espresso that morning—which was a good thing—considering how sternly we'd been warned against eating or drinking.

Walking in the door meant crossing the threshold into a lower energy vibration. The air seemed slower. Most of the people had friends or family with them; I had a magazine.

I got curious, sidelong glances, but I did not feel isolated or alone. I knew what I had within me. My children's kisses still lingered on my lips and cheek. My husband's confident eyes rested in my heart. I had already filled out all of my registration material, but I still had to sign in and wait.

In the middle of the room stood a podium with a little light shining down on a clipboard. At the front desk, a few feet behind the podium, a nurse shuffled papers. I'd already done my paperwork, so I was confused about what to do next. The shuffling paper nurse didn't look up. The podium's light still seemed to beam for attention.

Was I supposed to sign in? No one was in attendance there. Why did they use the podium? They actually needed a person to direct traffic with a little orange cone. This double sign in thing seemed silly. But we all did it. Did we really have a choice?

Signing in and waiting would shape my routine for the following year. Hurry up, sign in, and then wait. I had to come to peace with it. It was the hospital's routine. It was their language.

One man waited with his mother. She was the patient, but he was the one showing patience. Another man waited with his wife and child, and it appeared their child was the reason they were there. She was still in jammies, and I longed to join her. I had not showered that morning. We had been instructed not to wear any perfume, no hair spray or gel, no deodorant, no jewelry—not even a wedding ring or wristwatch.

In some way, this stripping down of our personality equalized us all. Up until this point, I had only experienced this sort of *class*, or *social* equalization, in two arenas, my church and my yoga studio. Now, dressed in the required loose-fitting clothing, all grooming aids and jewelry gone, we sat there, a group of strangers equal in waiting, for our lives to be altered.

One by one, patients were summoned, then passed through a corridor, never to be seen again. The room was emptying. Finally, the shuffling-paper nurse called my name. She asked, "Do you have someone with you who can help you through these initial steps?"

Initial steps? Were they planning on drugging me now? Did I need someone next to me while they weighed and measured me?

"No," I admitted. Defensively I added, "Michael is driving the carpool this morning." It was then 6:15 AM.

The shuffle paper nurse looked at me and I saw pity and skepticism in her eyes, a balloon over her head with words in it, *Sure, lady. Poor thing. She's all alone and can't even admit it.*

I planted my left hand on the desk. They'd made me leave my wedding ring home, but the line of white, untanned skin proved something, didn't it? She didn't seem to notice it.

Okay, I am a dork.

She motioned to another nurse, or maybe she was a nurse practitioner, or doctor's assistant, or teacher's assistant. Frankly, I wasn't in any shape to keep all their titles straight. I was just hoping that I would find Dr. Blumenthal at the end of the assembly line of scrubs.

My next nurse was wearing basic-blue hospital scrubs. He handed me a plastic bag and a whitish hospital gown. "You'll need to remove all of your clothing and put it and your identification here."

I had only my license and insurance card with me. The basic blue scrub nurse made me a hospital bracelet which duplicated my patient number and name from my file and placed it around my wrist. Every time I saw a new scrub, my ID bracelet would get embossed again with a small machine process.

I obeyed and put on the bleached-out gown. Now I looked like every patient who passed through the corridor.

I handed over my plastic bag.

The basic blue scrub nurse asked, "Do you have someone who can help you with these initial steps of surgery?"

The same question. The same identical tone of professional concern. I had the same response; defiant.

How pathetic I must seem. "Michael is driving our children's carpool this morning. He will be here shortly."

I received the identical pitying, skeptical look.

The basic blue scrub nurse turned me over to the IV nurse, whose scrubs fit her too tightly, in my opinion. She duplicated the bracelet, then asked me, "Do you know what your blood type is?"

Of course, I knew what my blood type was. I'd only heard that information a hundred million times over the course of last week. While I rummaged around in my brain, I glared at her.

"You just stuck a twig-size needle into my arm. Don't you know?"

She stared back, her face a total professional mask, but there was just a hint of, "Don't mess with me, lady. I have needles."

I stopped glaring.

She asked, "Don't you have someone here who can provide support during these initial steps?"

I drew in a big breath. "He has our kid's carpool this morning," I paused. "I asked him to take them to school."

She wasn't listening.

I stopped talking.

I was passed on from the IV too tight scrub nurse, out of the clothing removal room, to the sea foam, neon green scrub nurse, whose Filipino accent was so thick I couldn't tell if she was complimenting or insulting me. But she gave me the best gift I could have asked for. As we walked down another deserted corridor, we passed a deep-freeze unit. She lifted the lid and pulled out a blanket. When she handed it over, I was startled to discover that it was a warm blanket.

What a fantastic idea! What a beautiful, fantastic idea! This was precisely what my body and spirit was craving. As I clutched it to me, I suddenly realized I was shivering. It was just nerves. Even in my show my behind gown, I wasn't actually cold.

"Thank you." I said gratefully.

The sea foam, neon green scrub nurse smiled, then the look of professional concern took over and, in her thick accent, she asked, "Do you have anyone here who can be with you through these final steps leading up to your surgery time?"

I looked straight back at her and lied, "No." It was simpler than explaining.

She said nothing, simply took me into a room where a woman was waiting. Odd. She was wearing clothes. Office going clothes. She told me to lie down on the bed, "On your back."

I did.

"Wait just a few minutes, and your doctor will be in," and she left.

Ooooh! Perhaps someone I know?

Sure enough, my radiologist, Dr. Clark, entered the room. He greeted me warmly, "So, how is my runner?"

I tell him that I have clearance to continue with my plans to run the marathon, now just one month away.

He smiled. "Atta-girl!"

He injected several dyes and serums, explaining what he was doing and why. I retained no detail beyond observing that the color was blue. What I didn't know was that I would be seeing this color again fourteen hours later, as I threw up, over and over, giving new meaning to the verb "retch."

Then HE did the unthinkable! "So, do you have anyone here that can help you through this?"

I'd been willing to cut the other scrub ettes some slack. They didn't know me. I didn't know them. I had no interest in knowing them. What had they done for me, besides give me a warm blanket and plunging a needle into my arm?

But here was Dr. Clark, someone I actually knew. Someone I respected. Tough. I had to dock him some points.

"Michael, my husband." Dr. Clark had never met Michael. He came with me during every single prenatal visit during both pregnancies, and as I was about to discover, would take vacation days and sick days to attend every single chemo session so that I would not have to endure fear and illness alone.

Michael was being a proper father by taking care of our children and carpool responsibilities while I walked through the forms, the halls, the endless variations of scrubs before surgery.

"Michael is driving the carpool this morning. He'll be here soon." I could hear the insistence in my voice. "Really! Really! I swear he is!"

I must have been the most pathetic creature in the hospital. Alone. Breast cancer. Alone. Pretending she had a husband. Poor thing. There may have been a couple intervening scrub suits; but, finally, Dr. Blumenthal showed up. She asked where Michael would be waiting after my surgery.

Finally, an intelligent question! "He'll be in the waiting-room until you come out to see him."

She nodded. She believed me!

Just before entering the operating room, I said, "I'm a little nervous."

"I'd be worried if you didn't express these feelings," she assured me. "You're going to be fine."

They didn't tell me surgery was going to feel like torture. I had no idea that my arm was going to be strapped to a board. I could feel the anesthesia burning up my arm from the needle in my wrist. I felt panicky about being restrained, and doubly panicked because the mask covered my nose and mouth, preventing speech. I think surgeons do these procedures so frequently that they sometimes forget how terrifying it can be in its newness – how terrifying in its pain.

I remember making a mental note. *Remind Dr. Blumenthal that she should tell her patients about this step!*

But what should she tell them? To ignore it? To forget it? How do you remember to forget without remembering? When Oliver Wendell Holmes Sr. coined the word *anesthesia,* this is what he meant, *a reversible lack of awareness.*

I remember thinking, *I don't need to remember this part. This is not useful for me.*

That's the last thing I remember until I woke up several hours later. Leaning over me was Dr. Blumenthal, her expression just as professional as it had been when she first told me I had breast cancer.

"The lump was larger than we expected, Amy," she said. "It involves the lymph nodes."

She was going to talk to Michael. I'd be moved soon.

I didn't hear where I was going. I could hear a nurse in the background sternly instructing a patient to lie still, but I couldn't quite untangle Dr. Blumenthal's voice from the nurse's.

"You're probably feeling a little nauseous," Dr. Blumenthal said. I felt a lot nauseous.

She was going to talk to Michael, right?

I made my tongue work enough to say, "He was driving for our carpool this morning. He's in the waiting room."

I actually had no idea where he was. I, after all, had been unconscious for the last two hours.

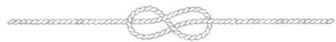

Dr. Blumenthal found Michael and explained the specifics. "You can see her in about forty-five minutes. We just wanted to be sure she's stable before we move her to her room." Michael had decided to move the car to avoid the parking police.

The nurses were ready to move me and apparently went out to the waiting room, looking for my husband. He was nowhere to be seen. They came back and began rolling me down the hall. I heard one of them say, "Poor thing! She must be delusional."

I squeezed my eyes shut.

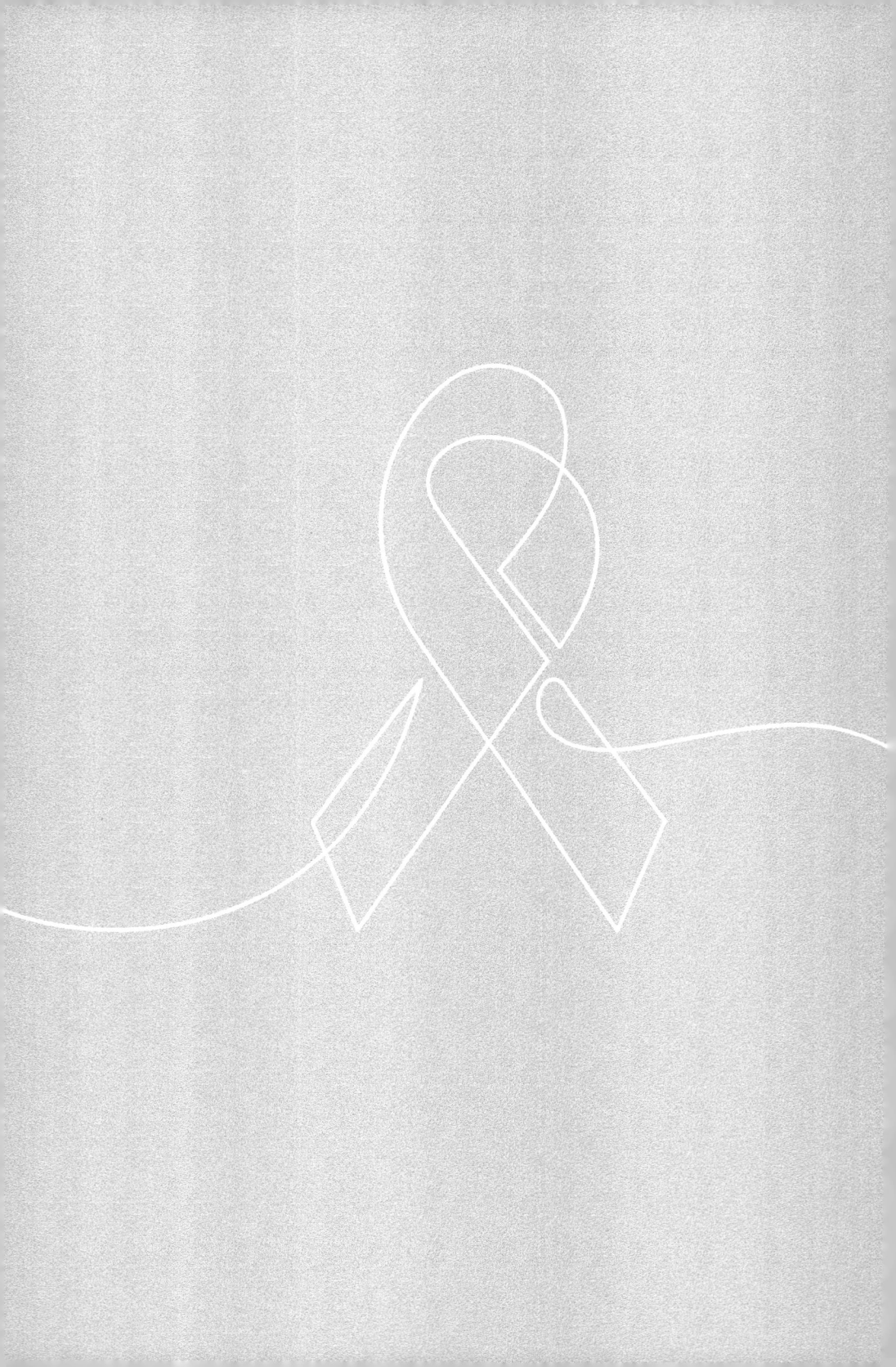

Telling People

When you put yourself wholeheartedly into something, energy grows. It seems inexhaustible.

– Helen de Rosis

Telling the people we loved about the cancer was harder than hearing the news for the first time ourselves. But a month later, after the surgery, we had already processed the information and had developed a game plan. Our friends and family had not had this luxury. Setting the schedule for disclosure patterned itself from the chemotherapy and the physical changes that would follow. We found that it needed to be contextualized.

We slowly became accustomed to telling our news to people that we know and love. Our instinct to wait, to draw in our resources and guard our privacy in those first days after the diagnosis, turned out to be sound. People diagnosed with cancer often become caregivers when announcing the news.

I would ask Michael, "How many people did you make cry today?"

"Three," he would announce somberly.

We started with our families. My mother, also a breast cancer survivor, took the information well but didn't like how long we had waited to tell her.

I explained that it wasn't about her, it was about us. We needed to have information. We needed to be able to direct people in a way that would be helpful for us. She got this, and I was grateful.

As a survivor herself, she immediately started networking with her friends and with other survivors. Soon I was receiving letters, gifts, care packages, and emails from all over the West Coast, Mexico, and Canada. Each message provided me with a loving touch.

A very wise soul told me in the beginning stages of telling, "This is not your time to be a martyr, Amy. Let people be part of your wellness plan. It helps them as much as it helps you."

So, we did. And yes, it helped—more than we could ever imagine.

We actually had two game plans. One was the *medical plan*, and the other was the *wellness plan*. Some helped with one, some with the other.

Each plan had a three-step approach.

(a) Gather information.

(b) Analyze it.

(c) Implement it.

The criteria were specific. It had to be workable, include others, and keep life feeling *normal* which required a fair amount of creativity. It would all result in a *new but used* me.

For the medical plan, the triad of decision-makers consisted of me, Michael, and my doctors. My surgeon, oncologists, and radiation therapist. When the treatment included medical intervention, the triad would discuss it, weigh the odds, make well-informed decisions, and then follow through with full commitment and full heart.

Michael carried a black book wherever we went. When we had a question, we wrote it in this book. He also wrote down answers, usually gathered in the doctor's office. That was his job. My job was to give my physicians my full attention.

This way, I was allowed to experience emotion. Frustration and tears, laughter and sarcasm, anger and determination.

I feel fortunate that a path had been cleared for me—even the medical plan. Before I left one doctor's office, the next appointment was set up. I was guided from one excellent physician to the next.

Initially, Dr. Anna Beck was my oncologist. In making this request, I was very pleased that she was able to make room for me in her heavy patient load. My knowledge of her was not personal but peripheral. Dr. Beck had treated my daughter's godmother, Jean. Jean only had marvelous things to say about her treatment as a person first and then as a patient second. This was important to me. I needed to be seen as a whole person, not just as a hospital I.D. bracelet to be duplicated.

What I loved best about Dr. Beck was the trait she shared with Dr. Blumenthal—their ability to simply be present with us.

I find this trait to be rare among physicians these days. My brother is a surgeon and has actually been reprimanded by his hospital for spending too much time with his patients. Ridiculous! During these initial office visits with Dr. Beck, a slow unveiling of our roles took place. Part of her role, as a physician, was to educate us to the protocol of treatment, beginning with Adriamycin and Cytoxan treatments semimonthly for the next two months. Followed by two more months of Taxol every other week. After Chemo, I'll receive daily doses of radiation for six weeks.

Michael documented everything in his black book. He is the kind of man that actually reads the instructions to everything before using it or putting it together. As a result, he is able to understand the mechanics of how almost everything in the universe works! I am an experiential kind of gal. I take bits of information from a variety of resources and put them together to see what comes up. I don't always meet with success, I've had a few explosions in my life thus far, but I always discover something new!

As Michael busily writes down medications, time frames, doses and side-effects, I am freed-up to infer what Dr. Beck wasn't saying, "Take care of your whole body. Don't let cancer run your life. Talk with your children. Take one day at a time."

The balance, the yin-yang, between Michael's and my approach to meeting with our doctors assisted us in our steadfast application of facing and living life with cancer.

Dr. Beck is someone we trusted implicitly and her advice to take charge of my life (and my hair!) was the message she infused in both of us. She set the foundation for us to build on, and I will be forever grateful to her.

My *wellness* plan involved another trio. Me, Michael, and my alternative medical providers. The owner of the health food store helped to educate me on me. He was able to guide me toward books on nutrition, vitamins, and homeopathic remedies that supported me without contraindications to my western medical treatment.

"She needs it." I heard Michael telling his friend's wife. "Whenever she tells me that she is off to take a yoga class and we need to rearrange schedules, I do it because she needs it."

I had to balance the two modalities. Taking into consideration that my whole body was going to be affected by my chemotherapy, I was insistent in supporting the parts of it that were not sick. You see, I never felt sick from cancer.

I discovered it. It did not discover me.

I had it removed and now my doctors were simply trying to keep it away. In the meantime, I was compelled to honor the strength my body was demonstrating, and I did this with ingredients that it would crave, Omega 3 oils, DHA & EPA, Vitamin E, antioxidants and lots and lots of green tea to keep me alert and happy.

When the treatment included acupuncture, homeopathic remedies, massage, vitamins, yoga practice, meditation, hiking through the mountains with our dog, Mazzie, or completing the marathon, the triad would discuss it, and the community of supportive and loving friends would make it happen.

I received my chemotherapy infusions at the Utah Cancer Specialists Corporation. It is not a huge building, and the philosophy governing it was personalized, step-by-step educational treatments. The staff expected and encouraged Michael and me to ask questions, discuss them, and compare chemotherapy approaches.

Chemo class was another great invention—right up there with the warmed blankets. We had to take this class before we started chemotherapy. A seasoned nurse met our class with an air of confidence and hope. She began by acknowledging emotions that we may be feeling.

"You've seen all the movies . . ." I remember her beginning.

Immediately, my mind raced through scenes from *Love Story*, with Ryan O'Neal and Ali McGraw.

"Well, a lot has changed since 1970!"

There were ten in our class. Not all of us were patients and not all of us were first-time cancer survivors. In this class I understood what determination really looked like. One woman, whose cancer had returned, was making second rounds of surgery, treatments, and recovery.

Our nurse expressed her feelings behind the strength of her patients but was sure to include the strength of her nurses as well. Our medical industry is such that patient's information requires protection. Our nurse was careful to keep anonymity regarding our specific cancers and treatments but was able to gracefully weave around the HIPPA laws to give us the information we were seeking. She explained the drugs in detail with us, describing side-effects and alternative methods to counteract them. She presented some tricks of the trade handed down to her by patients and fellow nurses. She even had information on where to find wigs and hats.

Amazingly, Utah Cancer Specialists also maintained a wellness calendar offering free services like massage, fly fishing, and Friday barbecues. I loved this idea! But I'm a pseudo-vegetarian, so a Friday ice cream may have suited me better, but still, I loved the wellness approach just the same.

I felt guided to the *right* people. Those I trusted, who had a reputable practice, and people with whom Michael and I felt compatible. We worked together on both the wellness plan and the medical plan.

Part of my infusion routine consisted of blood work, getting weighed, *never fun*, taking temperature and blood pressure, and ending with an escort to a private examining room where we wait for our doctor.

Halfway through my entire treatment protocol and just prior to the routine check-up before my next infusion, Dr. Beck softly announced that she was leaving Utah Cancer Specialists. I could tell that she was hesitant in making this disruptive announcement but had chosen her timing wisely.

For a moment, my mind interpreted her hesitancy as bad news. But, in the end, her news was anything BUT bad. We had come to know through our visits that she had struggled to balance her busy medical practice and being mom to two daughters in their early teens. She had been planning on semi-retiring for over a year; and when I chose to delay my treatments due to the marathon, well, this bumped my chemo schedule back one month. Thus, her transition came in the middle of my series of eight transfusions instead of at the end. By that time, we had experienced her integrity and patience so thoroughly that we understood and accepted her decision. She was choosing her family's A Quality Life Community. We understood that language.

She told us about Dr. Chandramouli. She quipped, "If you can't remember his name, think *guacamole*."

We remembered his name. He is of Indian descent, and he

took my wellness agenda in stride. He wanted to see a list of the vitamins I was taking but eliminated nothing from the list. He gave me research on the positive effects of Omega 3 oils, not only in supporting the effects of the chemotherapy but also helping to support the healthy parts of my body. I find EPA and DHA valuable even today.

I worked with my yoga teachers, Dawn and Kim, in guiding my breath and meditation toward empowering the parts of me that are still in working order. Then I could use these parts to help the "me" that was feeling compromised.

We wrote our questions down in our little black book. We looked for answers. I continued to train for the second biggest race of my life. I let people help me, and I listened to Michael.

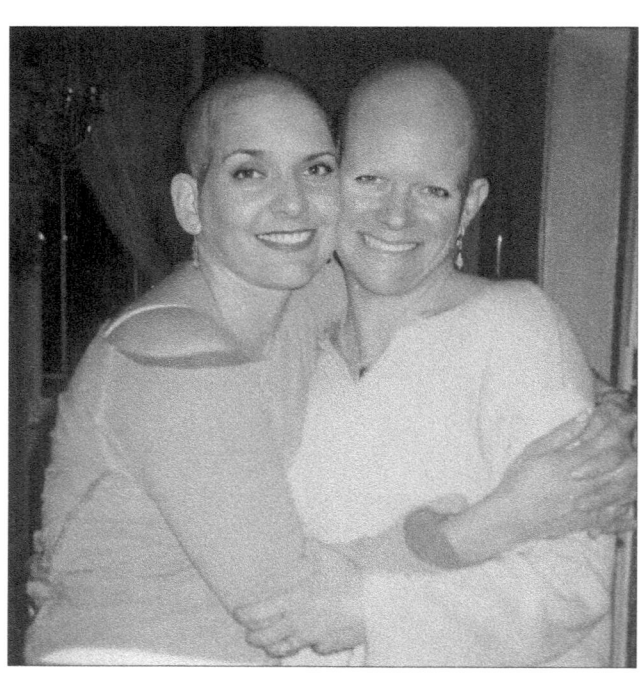

The Bald Party

*It is not joy that makes us grateful;
it is gratitude that makes us joyful.*

—Brother David Steindl-Rast

Michael, my husband and best friend, went first. He wouldn't have missed attending out of *shear* support—and the tequila, of course. When Michael's skull emerged from under his brown curly locks, we compared the results critically. I had decided that my head-shape would better suit baldness than would Michael's. His firefighting buddies already called him *Bert,* after the Sesame Street character with the long rectangular face. Baldness would only make Michael's head look more rectangular.

Would I fare better in the hidden scars department? I stared in surprise at a jagged *Harry Potter* lightning-bolt, pink scar on the back of Michael's head. "How did you get that scar, honey?"

"I was about eight years old and had two cats who liked to sleep on my bed. One day, they were each sleeping on opposite ends. I decided it would be a good plan to jump in just the right spot, somewhere near center, to make the cats pop up."

Everybody was listening, grinning, and anticipating that this story was going to end just awful.

"My idea was that the cats would shoot up from the bed and actually pass in mid-air, then plop down on the other end. It was a great plan! The only problem was, I had forgotten that this was the bottom bunk. So, I jumped on the bed, and jammed my head against the metal frame of the upper bunk! Blood squirted everywhere."

Everyone winced in sympathy.

Obviously, Michael had survived just fine, but I couldn't stop myself. "What happened next?"

"Mom was twelve doors down at the neighbor's, having a cigarette. My sister, Pam, called the neighbor. She was hysterical, but the neighbor told Mom that I had just bumped my head."

Michael was the youngest of four, and the only boy, so his mother had developed a less intense concern for his health than she had held toward her previous children.

"My mom took her time walking home. When she finally arrived, she met me covered with blood and trying to calm down my sister Pam." He paused with a smirk.

I was trying to count the stitches running along the puckered scar.

"Eight," he said before I could finish.

Everybody picked up a glass, and the stories kept coming, childhood memories about hair, disaster, and survival. More and more people turned their heads to the shears that night.

This party was a response to my oncologist's suggestion, "Take control of the hair loss. Shave your head," she advised me. "If you don't take control of the cancer, the cancer will take control of you."

I was a forty-four-year-old mother of two young children, I decided right then and there to do exactly what my doctor suggested.

I telephoned my friend Tina and invited her to my *Going Bald Party*. She was a blessing, scheduling play dates for my kids and organizing meals following chemo sessions. But this step took the whole cancer adventure to another level. Cancer was not going to be invisible anymore. Before, I could hide the drainage tube and the scar under loose tops, but not baldness. Even without chemo-induced menopause, I didn't tolerate heat well; the idea of a wig, July sunshine, and hot-flashes was too much. Bald would have to be beautiful.

I could hear some hesitant sorrow in Tina's voice, but I wouldn't go there. This was going be bald with a bang—tequila, beer, and food. Tina was beginning to get into it.

The idea was that we'd all shave our heads! The guest list grew. Family, of course. Friends who were almost family, and some, simply friend friends.

"I'm going to have a Bald Party—eating, drinking, dancing, and we'll all shave our heads. You can too!"

Which friends would say, "Great idea, Amy! What time?" Which ones would say, "Who's this again?"

I considered my children's reactions. My seven-year-old son Benjamin enjoyed a good party. He'd be okay. The key was my own attitude. I showed no apprehension. If I embraced baldness with the same level of acceptance as surgery, Benjamin and I would both be okay.

With four-year-old daughter Abigail it was different. She woke up crying one night, while party plans were in full swing. As we cuddled her, she sobbed, "I cannot have a bald teacher. Ms. Terry cannot be bald, too. All of the kids will laugh at me. I have bald parents, but I cannot have a bald teacher."

At the time, our children attended a cooperative preschool where parents had to volunteer for a number of hours per week. Terry, a gifted teacher, had taught Benjamin for two years and was in her second year of teaching Abigail, so she knew our family well. She was used to getting calls at home.

"Terry," I announced, "We need to come up with a lesson plan about hair, and we need it for tomorrow."

Terry listened, asked a couple of questions, and instantly devised a plan to alleviate Abigail's terror of being surrounded by the bald adults she would have to explain to her friends. Terry swooped through her house, seizing photos of herself with various lengths of hair, which she would show to the children the next day, as a lesson that hair-length doesn't change the basic person.

Michael assisted by suggesting a short cartoon about a jack-a-lope and a sheep who gets sheared. The sheep is embarrassed to show his pink hide, afraid he'll be laughed at. But the wise jack-a-lope tells the sheep that he has a *pink kink in the way he thinks*. Instead, he needs to look at life from a different perspective.

You need to lift your foot up and slam it on down,
and bound, bound, bound and rebound!

The cartoon ends with the sheep hopping and dancing across the desert, as his sheep's wool begins to grow again.

The children loved the cartoon, as they did Terry's show-and-tell of her growing and shrinking hair. They could see, in each photo, the obvious fact that she was always, still, Ms. Terry.

Then, Terry asked them the question, "If very short hair is okay, then wouldn't no hair be okay, too?"

The circle talks which followed among these wise four- and five-year-olds touched my heart. The children would cover their hair with their hands, inspecting the results in the mirror. They would face across the circle at children facing them, and say things like,

"I think I look pretty good."

"I don't look funny at all."

"Look! Ms. Terry, if I cover all of my hair, you just see my face. I like my face."

That was the end of Abigail's night-time sobbing over baldness.

There were twenty of us, the newly bald, by the time the

The Bald Party

evening ended. Family, fellow firefighters, and friends. At the party, Terry announced that she was going to grow her hair longer for *Locks of Love*, a charity that provides wigs for cancer survivors (locks of hair have to be a minimum of seven inches long). She also swept up the hair from the floor after everyone had been cut, clipped, and shaved.

I was neither the first nor the last, but when I took the stool, a silence fell on the laughter and storytelling. Nothing needed to be said. It was simply the reason of our gathering on that rainy evening in the garage.

Merb, my hairdresser, did a superb job, giving me a nice clean cut, and then an even better shave. And, some saving grace, my head shape was, indeed, more aesthetically pleasing than Michael's.

Then, when Merb was through with me, she unexpectedly exclaimed, "Oh, hell!" Handing me her razor, she demanded, "Your turn!"

Unsure, I inquired, "You want me to shave your head?"

"Yep!" she confirmed. "Now, pass the tequila."

Merb has the most amazing blue eyes, so large that they capture your attention immediately. Her eyes are the outward reflection of her heart. Bold, brash, and beautiful. I shaved her head bald that evening wondering about the implications for her future hairdressing referrals, "Try my hair stylist! The bald one."

Benjamin and Michael both have unusually lumpy heads. Somewhere Michael had encountered the science of phrenology—a way of identifying personality traits by the placement and size of skull-lumps. (Brigham Young, the much-married founder of Mormon Utah, is said to have had an enormous bump of *amativeness*.)

I looked up phrenological charts, and tried it out, feeling Michael's skull with my fingertips and palms, discerning enlargements or indentations to predict relationships and typical behavior.

Heck! Would it work for assessing prospective marriage partners? Or, as a background check for prospective employment? Could we raise grant money for a scientific study to see if firefighters—breast cancer survivors, too, have similar patterns of head-lumps?

It took about four months after chemotherapy and well into the radiation stage, for my hair to start growing back. Michael wasn't content with the one-time shave, he resolutely remained bald as long as I did.

He had about a dozen moles on the top of his head, another secret about his naturally hairy being laid bare. Every time he shaved, about every three days, he would emerge from the bathroom with tiny scraps of toilet paper sticking to each bloody spot. Although his technique improved with time, I don't think he ever survived a single week without loss of blood.

See why I love him?

Conversations on a Mountain Peak

The reasonable man adapts himself to the world; the unreasonable one persists in trying to adapt the world to himself. Therefore, all progress depends on the unreasonable man.

—George Bernard Shaw

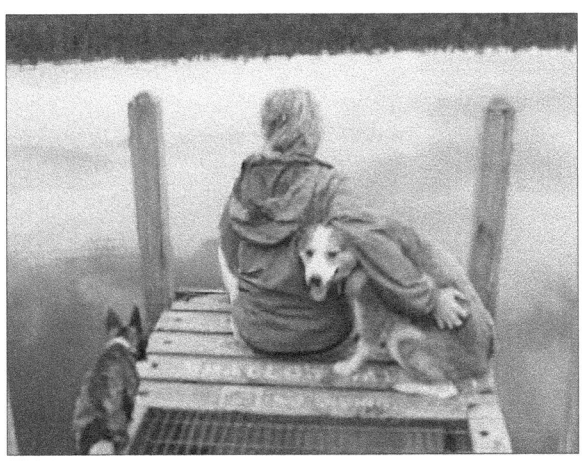

When I was first diagnosed, Mazzie and I climbed a lot of mountains.

I bargained with every chip I had, standing on whatever peak I reached that day, and I held fairly intense conversations with the clouds, the sky, and some fortunate birds who flew by.

With God and the universe.

I said pretty much the same thing each time.

"Okay, I understand I have some serious challenges ahead of me. If I promise to do what you want, will you give me forty-five more years? What do you want me to do? I have children to raise. They need me."

The trail up to the peak is a familiar one. Mazzie thoroughly enjoys running through the tall brown grass in the summer and tromping through nose-deep snow in the winter. I especially enjoy her forging her own path coming up only for air and, perhaps, view my location so as not to lose me.

We're companions on the mountain. On our hikes together we've witnessed deer with full racks cross our trail just twenty feet in front of us. Once, we spotted a cougar; another time a moose blocked our path cutting our hike short. On that particular day, the moose won. Often voicing my requests all along my mountain ascension, various wildlife became the ears for my desires. I imagined butterflies receiving my messages and flying them up into the heavens as little messengers for me and my mission.

I was bound and determined to seek what was wanted of me rather than discovering what was happening within me. But sometimes when I opened my mouth to start my daily bargain, instead of words, tears would come.

I finally realized that I was not pulling from my core where my strength resided. I was surrendering my power to fear. Fear of loss; of the family, of body parts, of purpose—climbing the mountain helped me face all of my primal fears.

One day, suddenly, my purpose became clear. I needed to combine the energy *around* me with the energy *within* me and draw from that source.

My mountain hikes continued, but instead of bargaining for more time, I reshaped my mountain peak conversations and turned them into progress reports.

"Things are going well. I feel a little alien in my body, but I am strong within. My frustrations about my body are dissipating and my fear is melting away. I'm eager to see what will happen next."

Gradually, everything in my life fell into place. My words, intentions, thoughts, and heart were finally acting from the same playing field.

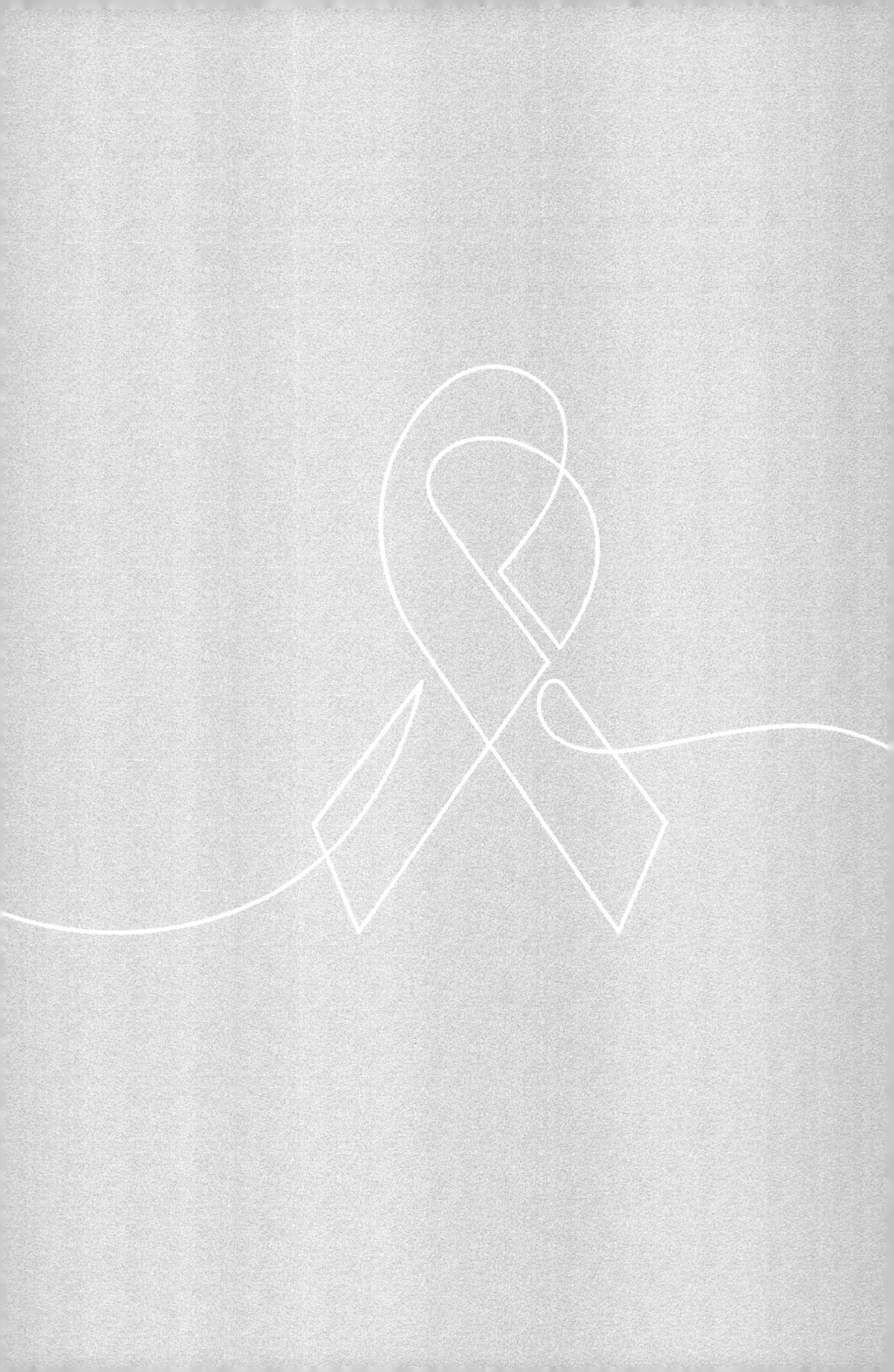

Five Bottles

Any time we catch a glimpse of soul, beauty is there. Any time we catch our breath and feel "how beautiful!" the soul is present.
—Jean Shinoda Bolen, M.D.

Most of my life I have struggled with *following directions*. Most of my report cards were marked with *N or Needs to Improve*. Typically, in the same two areas, *Listening thoughtfully*. (no surprise to anyone who knew me) and *Follows directions*. (I rebelled early)

I had tons of friends, however, I just found myself always pushing the envelope or crossing the line. I had this overwhelming sense of curiosity, so I would think outside the box, maybe the wrong box.

I wonder what would happen if I didn't do as I was asked?

I found it interesting that, although I still considered myself to be of a curious mind, the rebel in me would sit dutifully in the back seat while I did as I was told when it came to ordering my medications. I usually resist taking drugs that alter my state of awareness, but there I was at the Smith's Pharmacy window placing my order; and there were a lot of them.

I was so weary this particular evening that, even if the rebel in me had not moved out of the driver's seat, I think my fatigue of mind and body would have smothered my energy to act otherwise. I was listening and responding to the moment, moving purely from instinct. I was allowing my body to speak, and I was obeying. I handed the pharmacy tech my prescriptions.

At home, the kids were in bed and Michael was waiting for me to return. The sun of this 2005 spring evening was suspended on the horizon. I waited for my heart to make its next beat. I suppose I was seeking more something familiar.

It had been a long day.

Michael and I had taken on cancer as a second job. Our world had turned into a systematic management of several calendars; one now called the *Cancer Calendar*. I was told that I would have difficulty remembering details, so I wrote everything down. Again, I found myself automatically listening and following instructions.

I noticed the startled expression on the pharmacy tech's as she handed the prescription orders to the pharmacist. It was as if I had just handed her prescriptions that were written in a foreign language.

I was too tired to really care, but I noticed just the same. Experience teaches us that what appears may not always be what is. This tech didn't know me and what I'm capable of, I knew I could handle what was next. She only knew that my orders are consistent with someone preparing themselves to receive chemotherapy, but face must not have portrayed my bravery.

I knew they were just steps outlined by Dr. Beck, my oncologist. It was a well-reviewed prescribed protocol that Michael and I listened to and trusted, again and again. When the pharmacist glanced at the orders, she immediately became present, and she asked me to step to the other window, then she went about preparing my five prescriptions.

I probably didn't need them all, but I wasn't arguing right now.

Five Bottles

It's a funny thing to hear all of the sounds you miss when your mind fills the void of silence. There is so much sound in waiting, in patience, in presence; you are only aware of what is happening at each moment—nothing before, nothing after.

A row of chairs sat next to me, but I chose to stand. I'm not sure why. Perhaps I knew I would have fallen asleep if I didn't remain vertical. Maybe I was watching the pharmacist fill the order, checking and double checking each pill, each instruction. She appeared to be thorough, unhurried. Her body language communicated calmness. Her motions flowed from one sequence to the next, methodical, precise, undistracted, silent. Her job doesn't require much interaction with people. She prescribes nothing herself. She is simply fulfilling physicians' requests.

I didn't expect an interaction except for the simplest transaction. No relationship, no challenge, no interrogation for information. However, when she turned toward me with five bottles in her hand, she focused on me completely. She was explaining slowly and patiently. I hadn't started the treatment yet, but my ability to track instruction had already eroded. I strained to follow her interpretation of the directions.

"Take these the morning of Adriamycin and Cytoxan and these other pills following the second half of treatment. Take these when you're sad and these if you're nauseated."

I glanced out the window the sun had set; the sky outside was dark. I was alone with my pharmacist. I was struggling to make sense of this moment. My thoughts began to run wild while trying to internalize the instructions.

I'm a mother of two young kids. I'm happily married. I eat mostly vegetables and Omega 3 enriched foods. I'm in the middle of training for a marathon, and oh yeah—*I have cancer.*

It was too much. My eyes must have begun to well with tears, because she stopped, looked directly at me, and asked, "How are you doing?"

I told her that I was exhausted mostly. I told her that the whole experience was overwhelming and that I was doing my best to hold it all together. I told her I felt responsible. I felt that I needed to be calm but wasn't sure why. I told her that I was so tired. Could she possibly explain it again?

She could, and she did. She handed me the five bottles of medicine. I only needed the one my oncologist had said was not optional. The others were for the second half of treatment or as needed.

The pharmacist wrote her home telephone number on her business card and handed it to me. She said that if I ever needed clarification about any of my medicines, all I needed to do was give her a call, day or night. I heard this so clearly that it seemed to resonate throughout my entire body.

I've always considered Salt Lake City a small town with big city attributes. After all, it was a city that had a major university whose football team had just won the mountain west conference. It has four major hospitals within a stone's throw of our house and was big enough to host the winter Olympics.

But the small-town feeling keeps Michael and me here. We have found close communities within our city. This was the second time a friendly stranger in the medical field had handed me their home telephone number.

I never needed to call her, but I knew that I could. I was grateful for this moment.

Lists on a Whiteboard

Delight in the little things.
— Rudyard Kipling

My doctor gave us a *grocery list* of things to buy and a *to-do* list of things to complete in preparation for chemotherapy. It was helpful. It made this portion of the experience tangible, more concrete. It also gave us the sense that we could take control of some of what was happening to us.

Michael and I have always considered ourselves fairly simple people living in a complex world. We live fairly low-tech, we volunteer weekly at our children's school, we eat close to the earth, and we create things with our hands. When our oncologist suggested we buy a *memory board* (whiteboard) as a part of our grocery list and use it for simple messages and daily reminders, it was already a comfortable low-tech fit with how we conducted our lives.

Take morning vitamins.
Drink green tea.
Eat whole foods.
Walk every day.

These are simple, basic reminders. Did they really need to be written down? But Dr. Beck said we might be surprised about chemo's effects on memory and will. She also suggested placing the board in a central location, easily accessible. Michael placed it low enough so that Benjamin and Abigail could write on it, too, sending me daily reminders with little love notes and art creations.

Other list items were new to my life:

- Take two steroid pills the night prior to treatment.
- Take four steroid pills following each treatment.
- Continue for three days.
- Take anti-nausea pills for four days following treatment.
- Take anti-anxiety pills as needed.

Almost at once, Michael changed the order of the daily tasks on the memory board.

First and foremost, *"We love you."*

The memory board became a symbol of our new life for a while. It fit our simple lifestyle. It was tangible enough for everyone from age four to forty-four to manage. It also made cancer *not so scary*, as Abigail said.

Cancer, itself, is rather invisible to most people, but its effects conjure up the emotions that swirl and storm and slither around it. Michael and I spent so much of our energy simplifying it for our children that I think we ended up better understanding it ourselves. By discussing cancer in detail with Benjamin and Abigail, we could make this experience have some shape and sense for us as adults. The memory board ended up being a tool for this transference of meaning.

Was this Dr. Beck's intention? Was this a secret that she knew and wanted us to experience? She told us to *always be honest* with our children. "It makes it less scary." Abigail's words.

My doctor's words. She was right.

The memory board helped us take back our life.

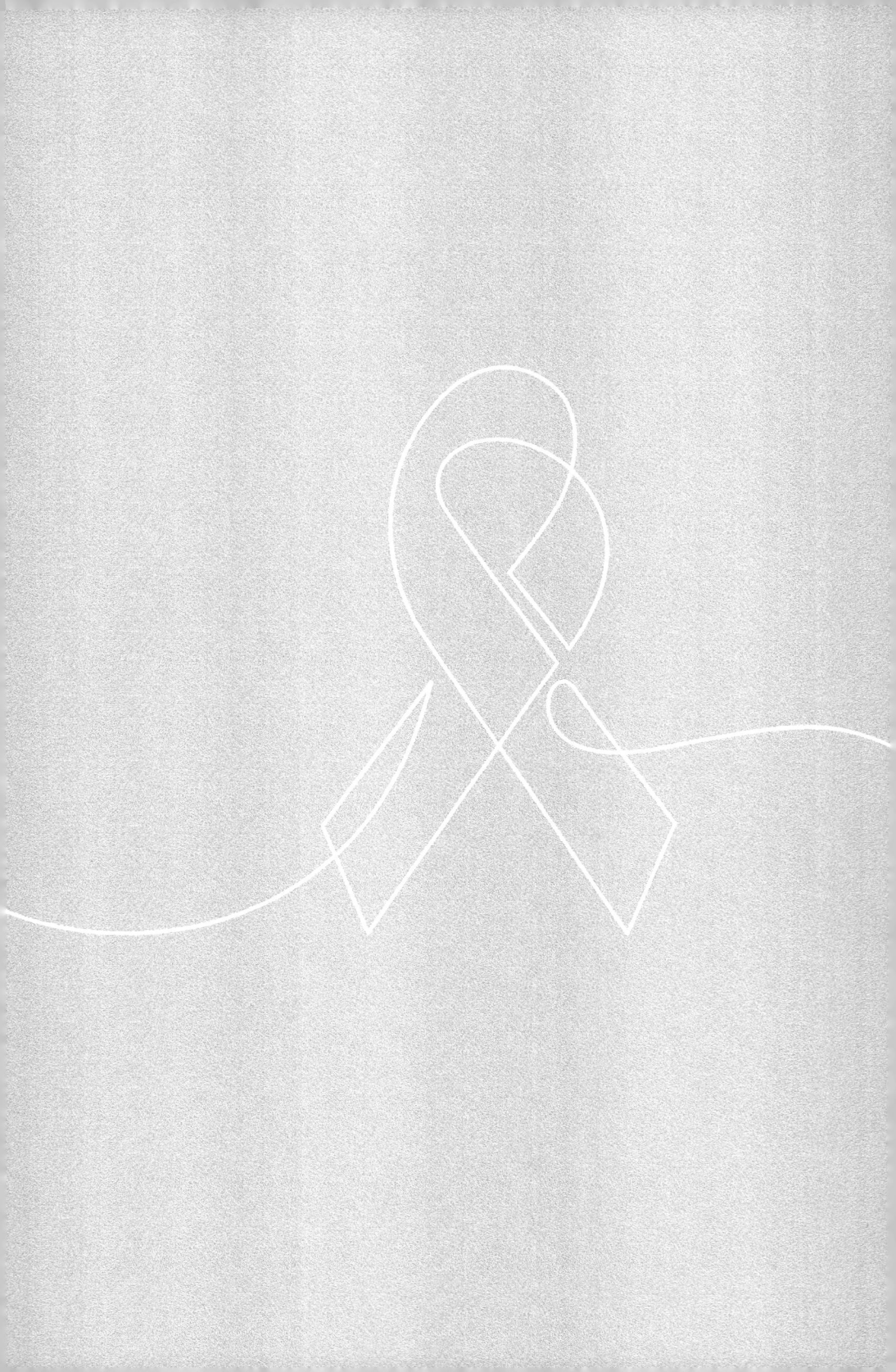

White Noise

The path to our destination is not always a straight one.
We go down the wrong road, we get lost, we turn back.
Maybe it doesn't matter which road we embark on.
Maybe what matters is that we embark.

—Barbara Hall

Like white noise, layers of thoughts, strategies to unresolved problems plans, ideas, and dreams. They run through my head, working in my favor most of the time but occasionally, against me.

"I can't sleep, I have so much to think about." I wiggle Michael awake to help me in my sleeplessness.

"Ah, well, stop thinking and then you can get back to sleep."

That seems logical.

What kind of a response is that? Not at all what I needed. It's the white noise in my head.

In making my game plan for cancer, I had to calm the white noise, focus on the issue at hand, eliminate the chatter of plans, ideas, worries, and impressions.

I would ask Michael again in the middle of the night, "Did I really put together our children's scrapbooks so that they could remember me?"

I had a path to clear. Cancer was an obstacle, not a result of anything I did, and the white noise during my late-night hours alone in a house filled with people needed to know this.

So, I meditated and practiced a lot of yoga.

Centering myself helped to center my direction. Once my mental GPS directions were input, the drive became almost—dare I say it—predictable? The obstacle became a hurdle, the hurdle became a speed bump, the speed bump a yield sign, which faded into through traffic and eventually onto the autobahn.

It required maintenance, however. Practice takes practice. Cancer became manageable, perhaps, because I thought of it as simply a cell gone mad. But the fear behind the cell accelerates the white noise back up to obstacle level again.

The solution?

For me, it's calming down the firing synapse to refocus on the matter at hand. Is cancer simply a cell gone mad? Or is it a lesson on how to live?

The Vice Patrol

*Always leave enough room in your life to do something
that makes you happy, satisfied, or even joyous.*

—Paul Hawken

I am now a born-again Dancing Leaves green tea drinker—two tea bags and sometimes over ice—always with honey. But is it really about the tea?

Chemo made me hypersensitive to my most beloved chemicals, wine, coffee, and sweets. I simply couldn't consume them. When I did, my heartbeat accelerated to thunder. I felt nauseated, sweaty, short of breath. Damn! With more and more being taken away from me, "Forbidden!" and "Not allowed!" I found my patience level decelerating. This body ban, however, extended to foods containing preservatives, but their exclusion wasn't catastrophic.

Being deprived of vices is a terrible loss.

I remember that, on one of my first visits to Utah Cancer Specialists, I was in the transfusion room chatting with all of the *hook-ups*—people connected to their IV trees. This experience always reminded me of a row of RVs plugged into their electrical outlets.

On one chemo visit, I'd had an allergic reaction, lost control of my bowels, and threw up my breakfast into a bowl held by one of my nurses. I quickly envisioned my particular model of RV visiting the sewage dump. It's funny what your mind travels through when it watches your body experience the *flight or fight* phenomenon.

In any case, one of the *hook-ups* had a cigarette vice. He would actually wheel his IV tree stand outside to have a smoke! I just kept thinking, "He's got chemicals dripping into his body so he can get rid of his cancer but he's outside smoking to be sure the chemo doesn't get it all!"

I had scheduled my infusion appointments during my lunch hour so as not to interrupt my teaching schedule. It was during this time that I discovered just how much of a loss losing my vices meant to me. Lunch hour in the infusion room at Utah Cancer Specialist was a lovely place for my olfactory senses but terrible for my taste buds.

Chinese food, Mexican food and huge ice cream shakes from Salt Lake's infamous Iceberg ice cream shop were bought by family members for all of the other hook-ups around me. I was surrounded by scent-sations that drove me wild and made my stomach churn for their meals. But alas, I knew that if I ate even a single bite, my heart would respond in a way that would make me feel ill. Resigning to my defeat to my vices would only be resolved with the acceptance that this, too, would be temporary and, once again, my patience was called upon.

I am grateful, however, that my vices were not all exclusive and, indeed, included some of the free samples distributed by Costco employees. I love Costco! I can spend hours walking through their stores; it's Disneyland for adults. I synchronize my shopping for the distribution times of free food samples. On occasion, these samples actually have veggie themes, which just thrills me. But no matter what's offered, I often sample enough to constitute a small meal. The problem was that some of these samples contained preservatives, sugar, or salt, and my body was saying. "No, no, NO!" My heart raced as I realized my defeat.

Chemo vs. Costco; chemo would always win. This was a terrible revelation for me.

When you're bald and being pumped up with steroids so your body doesn't reject the poison being infused into your body, suddenly, things like Costco samples begin to run your life. Dark chocolate offered a nice reprieve to my body rejection. High degrees of cacao made the food cut. Getting my next chocolate fix turned into an obsession. I correlate this experience to being nine months pregnant and knowing instinctively where every clean bathroom existed within the city limits of Salt Lake. I could have pinpointed them on a map.

Now I could switch those high-fidelity locating devices in my brain to track down stores that carried chocolate with high levels (75 percent and above) of cacao. I have since learned to just carry my own stash.

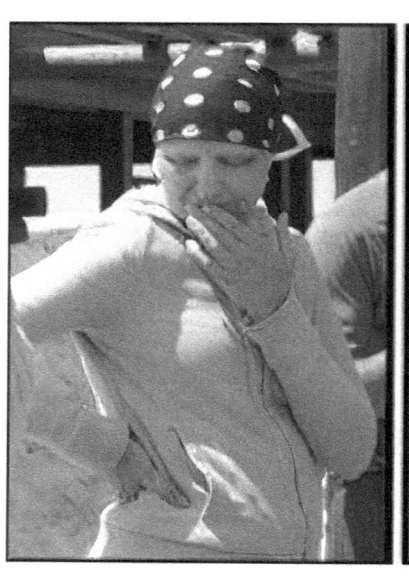
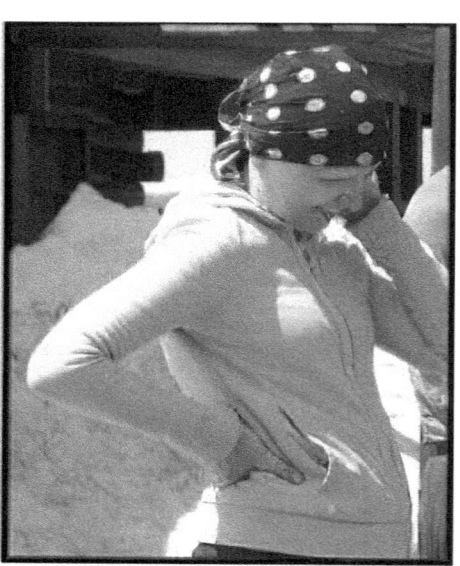

Kickback

*I said in my heart, "I am sick of four walls and a ceiling.
I have a need of the sky. I have business with the grass."*

—Richard Hovey

"I don't want to be poked anymore!"

My body was sending the message that it was tired of being abused. I can give it over to science for a while, but then I want it back. My body was on loan to the authorities to be their pin cushion, but this was not an open-ended arrangement.

Eventually, my veins screamed, "No more blood!" and shut down. No amount of hydration made them plump up. My veins somehow *knew*, even anticipated the next procedure. Somehow they became a separate entity with a mind of their own.

The solution was a port, another invasion, another intrusion. But I didn't want *another* surgery. My doctors told me that the surgery itself was considered minor, that it could be performed under conscious sedation.

However, my body screamed, "No more surgeries!" The truth was, I resisted anything that inhibited me from being physical. The port was a silicone bubble with an attached plastic catheter, which would be inserted under the skin in my upper chest with the catheter inserted into my subclavian vein. The port looks like a bump under my skin.

To my doctors, this procedure appeared to be an obvious solution to collapsing veins. A port is also a great device for nurses who administer chemotherapy; but the bottom line was this, I didn't want a port-a-cath. For me, I knew the port would interfere with my yoga practice; and at that moment, my practice was the one thing that kept me sane.

Were my doctors attempting to punch a hole in my heart rather than just a hole in my chest? Did they know that this was not the way to hurt me? Yet it would hurt. Did they know that this was not the way to heal me? Yet this was an option to deliver healing medicine. Despite the possibility of another hole, my body would not be deceived. I opted out of the port procedure with the agreement that if or when my veins completely collapsed, I would concede to a new hole with a whole heart.

My healing comes from deep within.

My body started to shut down in anger, yet it was my healing spirit that stoked the flame. In my mind, the doctors followed their protocol to keep me cancer free, but it was *my* job to keep me alive.

Eyelashes

When the body is weak, it takes over command.
When strong, it obeys.

—Jean-Jacques Rousseau

Hair growth has its own stages:
- Peach fuzz: not-quite hair.
- Spring growth: first hairs.
- *Fro* chemo curls. This stage lasts about a year.
- Awkward hair: half curly and half whatever the original hair follicle was before cancer. Also, the color of hair may change, thanks to the months of stress.

But that's hair on your head. Eyelashes are different. It didn't matter when someone told me that they would grow back. I held onto the one I had for as long as I could! I didn't lose my lashes and eyebrows until radiation had already begun, so I thought I was going to beat the odds everybody had warned me about during chemotherapy and keep my facial hair. After all, I still had to shave my legs, and I couldn't care less about that hair!

Then one day, I woke up and it was gone. My last eyelash! No longer would I need to spend minutes in front of the vanity mirror, painstakingly brushing mascara on my single eyelash. Laugh if you want to, but have you ever been bald on your face? Eyelashes took on a whole new meaning when they decide to go away.

My eyebrows were different. I'm a strawberry blonde, so I've never really *managed* my eyebrows. As a child, I was teased that I had none. When I went swimming, my skin tone and eyebrows blended into one. Usually, I forgot I had any.

Once I dyed them dark brown as an experiment. They were hideously conspicuous. Michael didn't really say anything, just smiled and cocked his head to one side. It was obvious he was waiting for my announcement indicating my tone so that he would know how to respond without causing me too much emotional insecurity.

"I've had some work done on my eyebrows," I blurted.

He was raised in the Midwest by a well-mannered mother, so he commented only, "Oh, really."

Another polite pause followed, but I was waiting for more.

"Well, they look nice."

I know when he's lying.

"Ummm, you know, natural looking."

"Do you think anyone will notice them?" I already knew the answer.

"Perhaps," he responded cautiously. "Do they—um—fade over time? Just asking! It's not like, you know, they need to or anything…"

"You hate them! They're ugly! I knew you wouldn't like them. They're like permanent pencil streaks tattooed into my forehead, and they won't come off!"

Now, I was hysterical.

Michael took my hand and said exactly the right thing, "I love you with or without eyebrows."

Well, I got to put this bold claim to the test. Not only did my last eyelash just fall out, but my brows had been thinning considerably. "They're about to jump ship any minute!"

My face is bald.

I tried to consider it an interesting experience. I'd gotten used to the newly exposed head shape. I had saved a fortune in shampoo and hair products. But facial baldness? I thought I looked like an alien—a human lizard.

"Is this a problem make-up experts can solve?" I continued my inquiry with Michael. "I'm already out of my body with all of the medical interventions. I'll need to stay as connected to being human as I can."

He listened.

My face is bald.

In one respect, I'd started with a clean slate to a new me, a new palette for a new face. I became a portrait that, even I, had not yet had the privilege to see. Perhaps this eyelash-less face was the best way to take the next step forward, into and through, my cancer adventure.

I was not a bald face, but rather, a portrait to be created on a new canvas.

Okay.

Big breath in, big breath out.

I was ready.

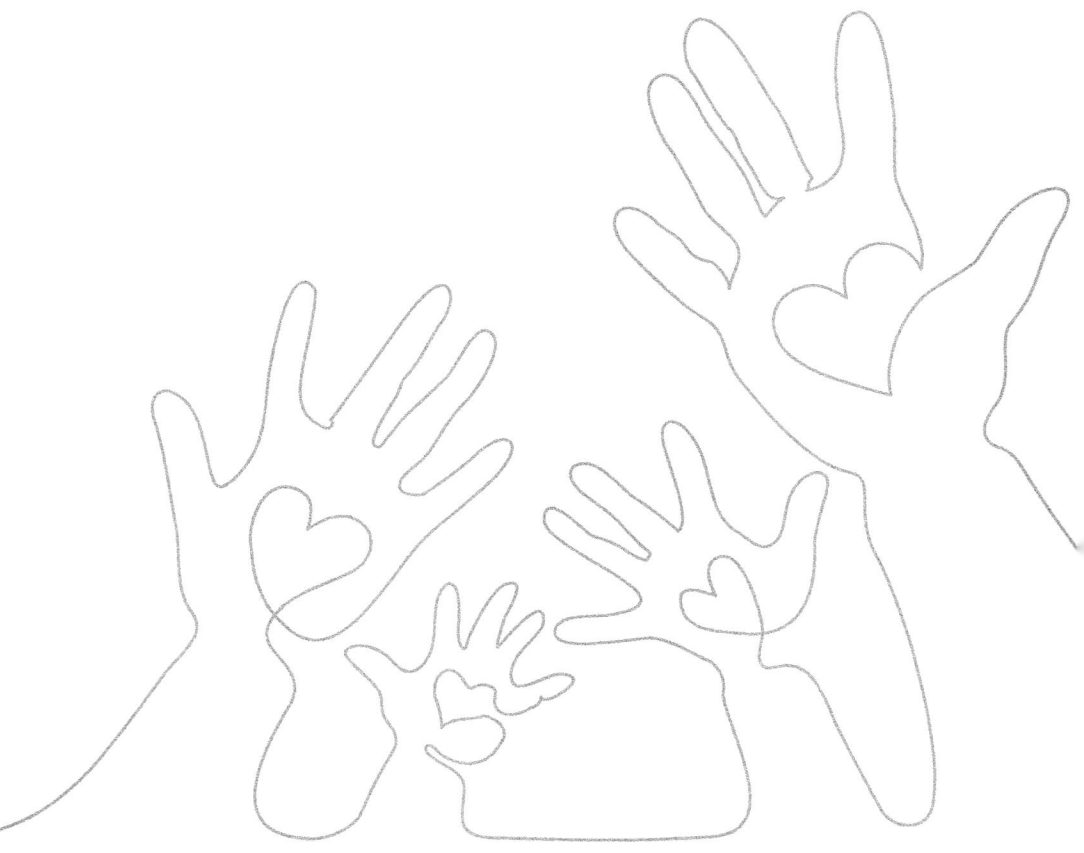

PART TWO
My Family

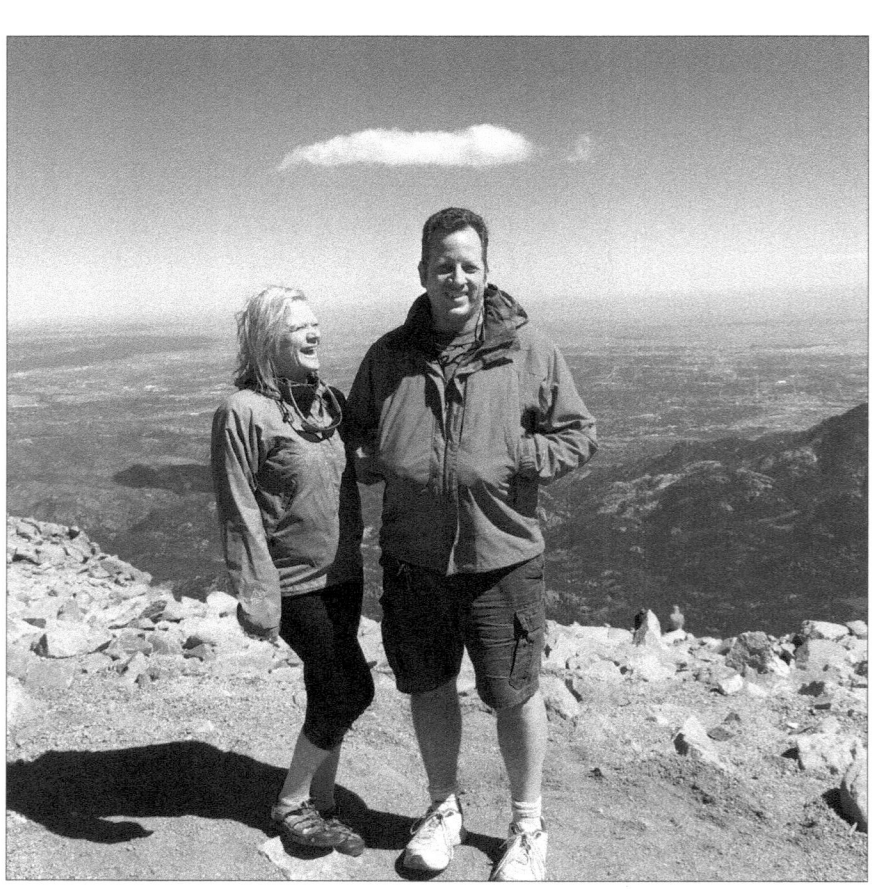

Meeting Michael

The best and most beautiful things in the world cannot be seen or even touched. They must be felt within the heart.
—Helen Keller

I've gone through life making a billion decisions, not always knowing what lay breath to any particular one. Sometimes, my decisions don't seem to lead me to where I intend them to. Then there are times when everything falls into place, and I find myself blanketed in gratitude for making those very uncertain decisions, because they led me to that place of welcomed grace, that loving place of balance and benevolence. Nevertheless, I've found that if my intentions were toward love, pure and simple, then, that's what I'll inevitably find.

When I was once looking for help, I found Michael, my husband—the love of my life. When I first met him, I was a high-school teacher for the Deaf and hard of hearing in California. As part of my curriculum, I introduced my students to one of my own great passions: rock-climbing. They weren't motivated by the typical teenage need for thrills or attention seeking. These were youth who needed—excuse the expression—a "crash" course in confidence. They had chosen rock-climbing out of a smorgasbord of choices, and they were all on-board to give it a go.

I had been turned away from three different rock-climbing gyms, and their instructors all reported back to me the same excuse, "We feel the *situation* causes too much liability."

I became more persistent. From my own experience with rock-climbing, I was well aware of its confidence-boosting benefits.

My students came from many cultures—one of these was being Deaf. More often than not, my students' parents never learned American Sign Language. Parents relied on their teachers and interpreters for all of their children's life lessons. I had Vietnamese, Laotian, African American/Cambodian, Taiwanese, and Hispanic students. Their parents spoke their native language at home. If they were able to, they would speak English when they were meeting me at school. Most parents saw deafness as a disability rather than a cultural difference.

This perspective on deafness, combined with traditions carried from their native countries, often left their children with poor self-esteem. By high school, that resulted in poor and uninformed choices.

One of my students was raped because she got into the car of a stranger who she thought he was good-looking and smiling. Another became pregnant, the result of much the same reason.

Two of my students were on the verge of getting kicked out of their homes, and all of this was linked to a lack of communication and education.

I managed to persuade all of the parents to sign permission slips so I could take them on a city adventure—climb a wall and build some confidence. It was my desire that this experience would eventually lead them to honoring themselves, which would give them the power to make better choices. The Deaf community was more than willing to cooperate with me. They assisted with organizing interpreters and even found experienced rock-climbing instructors who were also Deaf.

The hearing community gave me the most difficult time!

It was 1991; indoor climbing gyms, though on the verge of

becoming popular, were not yet abundant. My Deaf students were still considered a *challenging* group. The sport of indoor climbing was new, so were the rules that governed the walls. Furthermore, most supervisors and store owners did not know what the rules were.

I understood why they erred on the side of caution. I just didn't agree with them.

Michael's was the rock-climbing manager at the Sport Chalet in Huntington Beach, California. His position offered him some latitude for creativity.

For example, the typical placement for a wall was on the inside of the building, but Michael had designed a climbing wall on the outside of the building. The wall was enclosed in a fenced-off area in the back of the store and had nine routes with various degrees of difficulties. The climbing wall drew customers to the shop, making it a win-win situation for everyone.

Michael didn't hesitate when I asked about lessons for my group of students, instructors and interpreters. What he didn't tell me, until later, was that he had been taking sign language courses at the local community college.

We placed one interpreter at the top of the twenty-five-foot building, for when the climber/student would look up, and we placed another at the foot of the wall for when the climber/student would look down.

This triangulation enabled my students to climb, as well as communicate toward their desired direction. Because both signing and climbing require use of the hands, all students were "top roped," allowing them to let go of the wall and still be supported.

I like to find metaphors in everything, and this one was significant to me. I wanted my students to know, "You can let go of everything for just this moment in time and still be held up. We won't let you fall. We won't let you down. Tell us what you need."

The day was successful in many respects. It marked the

beginning of relationships that laid foundations for trust. I was able to take these same students to a YMCA Deaf Camp for five consecutive years following that first rock-climbing experience. I was invited to eat dinner with some of my students' families, who were often too poor to feed themselves adequately.

I felt honored and cherished to join them, in full Cambodian tradition, on a beautiful mat laid out on the floor of their apartment. Communication barriers persisted, too, but we ate in celebration of our shared belief that we simply must begin somewhere, and that eating food together was a way of sharing love.

In my pursuit for a rock-climbing facility for my students I met my angel, Michael. It was at least two months before I told him that I intuitively recognized him when I walked down the aisle of the sporting goods store—I knew I would be with him for the rest of my life.

I actually had the thought, *Oh, this is the guy for me!*

I fell in love with him immediately.

Three years after that rock-climbing Saturday afternoon, Michael and I were married. At our wedding, we included two interpreters, one for the male voice and one for the female voice.

The service was on the grounds of the Long Beach Museum of Art, overlooking the ocean. Catalina Island glistened in the distance. We exchanged our vows as the sun slipped into the ocean, before our friends, family, and students.

Our cake was the shape of a mountain, with bride and groom rock climbers, iron, welded by an artist friend. The groom, with welded top hat, was belaying his bride bedecked with a white lace train, to the top of the mountain.

During his toast Michael's best man, Mark, bestowed on Michael his own title of *Best Man*. He lifted his glass toward Michael, "There is no man better. A man who is willing to help, to support, to lift up…. it's just who he is, because it's the right thing to be."

And so, he is.

Michael's goodness is completely evidenced in his willingness to remain present. Regardless of sacrifices, he has never altered his commitment to remain present. That is my definition of a hero. I have been sure of this since the beginning of our relationship. We entered the cancer adventure as a unit, each present and ready to accept the challenge of the climb.

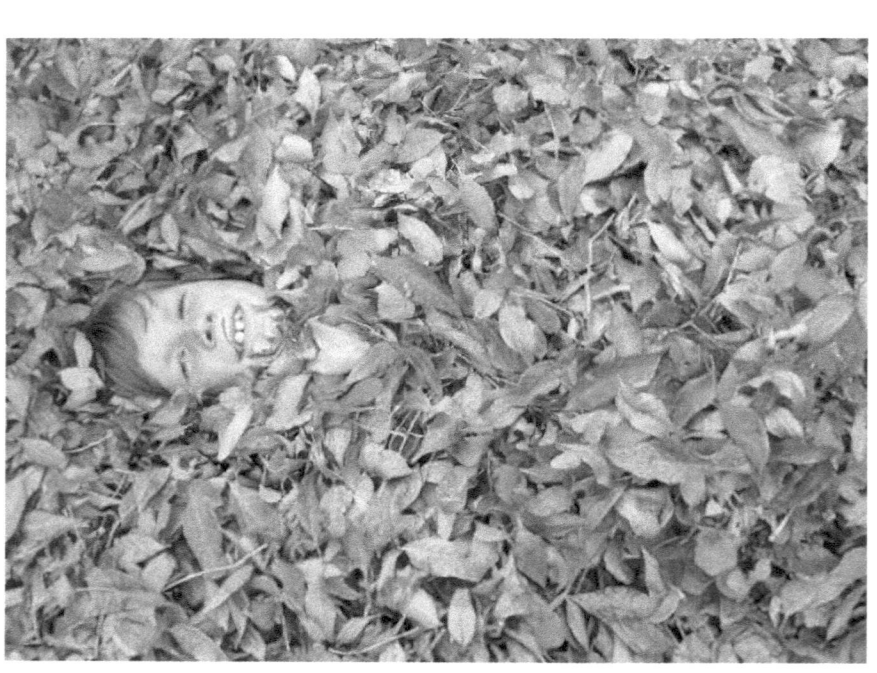

Benjamin's Window

From there to here, from here to there,
Funny things are everywhere.

—Dr. Seuss

When cancer found us, we were living in what I fondly called our *San Francisco house*. Our Salt Lake City home was an old one; built just twenty-five feet wide and forty feet deep. You could have a conversation with our neighbor through the bathroom windows. Thank goodness for our neighbor's San Francisco modesty.

We loved this house. We worked on the backyard for five years, making it comfortable for entertaining guests. We ate almost every meal there during the summertime.

Michael installed a misting system that lowered the temperature twenty degrees during the hot summer days and early evenings. We had an herb garden and a tomato garden.

We had a two-car garage with a workshop for Michael. We built a swing set with a fort for our children, and I had my rocking chair glider. This was all that I needed to watch the nature in the yard, feel the breeze, and listen to the sounds of my family. This was a great place!

One of my favorite spots in the house was my son Benjamin's room. The size of a large closet, we put a mattress on an elevated platform. Underneath was storage for his toys. Michael built a bookshelf with a bulletin board as a headboard. On the very top we built another shelf that held sweet treasure boxes and a night light that twirled around and projected stars on his walls and ceiling. I painted the ceiling of his room with clouds on a blue sky, and for night, I stuck glow-in-the-dark star stickers.

I painted a city scene with Michael's fire truck and his station number on it. I painted our home with our whole family, including Mazzie, the dog, and Mildred, the cat, standing beside it. It was three-year-old perfect. Benjamin loved this room and so did I.

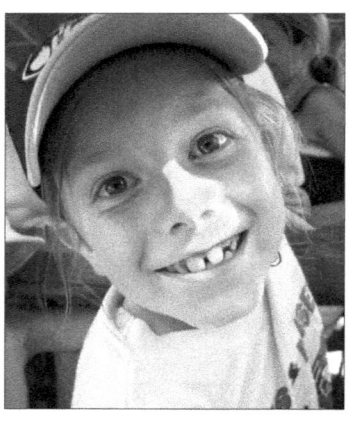

He had a small window, just two panes, that we upgraded so he could open it safely without any chance of falling out. The open window let cool air in and allowed him to lie on the edge of his bed watching the world go by. These were the moments that I loved best about my son's relationship with his room and his window.

When I asked him what he could see, he would say, "I see our neighbor across the street dancing in the rain. Sometimes I watch our neighbor's family play football on the grass island in the middle of the wide street. I see kids riding their bikes. I like riding mine. I see cars going by, and Mazzie running back and forth on the sidewalk in front of the house. I love the dragonflies best, Mom. They are spirits from heaven. I think they have chosen our house to fly in front of. I don't see them anywhere else. . . . They are like Snoopy and the Red Baron diving down and then zooming back up into the sky."

The window was very small, but, from Benjamin's perspective, it was the portal to the world outside. I loved watching the sunset fall on his face and his auburn hair as he watched the kids on the block turn toward their homes for the night.

Cancer and chemo occurred while living in this house. By the time I started radiation therapy in September 2005, we had moved to a new home in our new neighborhood.

Recently, I took Benjamin back to our old home and asked him to look at his window.

"Wow. It's so tiny!" he marveled, pointing up at the house.

"You lived in that room from the time you were three until we moved out when you were seven. You loved that room, do you remember?"

He nodded and added, "I remember Ben T. asking me, 'Is your mom okay? Has she grown any hair yet?' I remember that he would ask me a lot. He is my best friend and I think he was worried about me."

I could see that he was thinking about this time.

I get a little nervous about how different we looked when we left, since Michael and I were both bald.

But Benjamin is sharing his way of remembering. "It was funny having Dad have a bald head, too. Dad always makes funny faces. He crosses his eyes and does something funny with his mouth. I remember getting a black marker and drawing a face on the back of his head. Our friend, Lu, drew a sheep on the top of her head."

He's cracking himself up now. "I wanted you to have hair again, but not Dad. It was fun to draw faces on the back of his head."

"I remember you lost your mind for real, Mom."

He elbowed me in the ribs. "You had chemo brain and we needed to get you a board to remember things."

There was an aquarium at the cancer center that had a fish that looked like the absent-minded character Dory from the movie

Finding Nemo. "That was funny. Mommy was Dory."

He then started running lines from the movie with me. "Why are you following me?" Dory would ask. He laughed at himself. I laughed with him, because everything he says is absolutely true.

"I remember the dogs that would visit while you had tubes in your arm. I remember seeing other people getting chemo, too." He says these things, as if trying to make a connection in his own memory bank of experiences. I believe that if he can do this, then the memories will magically become *okay* for him.

"I remember when I got my tonsils out."

He was nine for that operation.

"It hurt like getting tubes in the hand—like what you got." He paused, then smiled, "Oh, yeah, and I got to ride in a wheelchair. That was awesome."

Cancer shifted all of our perspectives that spring, summer, and fall. Unexpectedly, we found a house that could fit our growing bodies that brought all our activities but Michael's fire station into one neighborhood. Our home was close to our school and also near my hospital. In addition, it gave Benjamin a larger window.

It's the house we still live in.

We moved when he was almost eight, and now his bedroom window has sixteen panes through which he sees sunrises rather than sunsets. Mountains, rather than street intersections. He can view the backyard and things that are private to him.

He tells me, "I'll be able to see the seasons change from this window."

His perspective seems to be more in balance with this new portal to the world. He tells me not just about what he sees but about what they mean—his interpretation of what the world is. "It's odd, Mom. A pleasant day can equal bad dreams and then a bad day can equal pleasant dreams."

How quickly he shifted.

It's been just a matter of months, but suddenly, I realize what lies behind his meaning, as if a horse's blinders were finally removed. Benjamin was saying that his view had widened—that he could see from a broader scope. I believe there was still wonderment and magic in his sight and in his mind, but he was no longer limited to just the differences of *what is* compared to *what can be*.

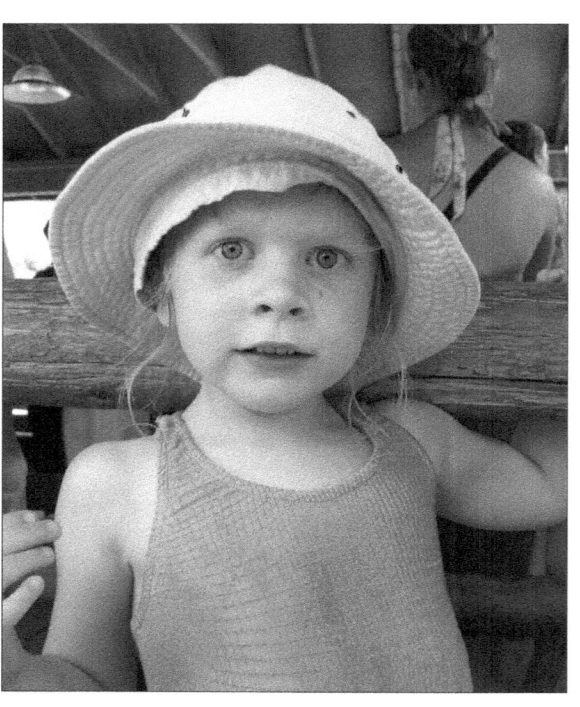

Abigail's Swing

Forget not that the earth delights to feel your bare feet and the winds long to play with your hair.

— Kahlil Gibran

When the world gets too noisy for my daughter, she retreats to her swing or to a rocking chair. She puts everything else on hold, then rocks it into perspective. Or perhaps she prefers to be part of the audience, not a participant. In either case, she has always done this, since the moment she could sit up independently.

Me, I'm a bouncer. I bounce against the backs of couches, love to rock in rocking chairs, and recall, as a child, the transition of outgrowing my swing set as being difficult. I loved my swing set and considered my time there a significant period in my life. Like Abigail, I loved watching my brothers and sister play. I liked being in the audience once in a while, not always interactive.

Swinging was my moving meditation.

Abigail can swing for hours at a time. It seems she needs to think, and this is her place.

She'll suddenly say, "I need to take a break, Mom,"

"Okay." I would have no idea what was jarring her world, but I understood her need instinctively. "Have fun. I'll call you when dinner is ready."

Moving backward and forward seems to help her mind open up to imagination, to the clouds, to the sky where her mind takes her body to fly. She loves watching kids play. She loves watching her brother entertain the other kids. She loves being the audience to his performances. Swinging is her moving meditation, too. It's a peaceful place for her to think. Seeing the good and feeling the peace.

Swinging, this movement of back and forth seems to have helped her cope with any perceived stress she may have experienced.

"I lose my mind," she told me once. "I feel like a cloud floating in the sky. When I look backward, it feels like I am flying."

When we were building a garage, and half of the swing set was is in pieces, Abigail frets. "I miss being on the swing."

One summer night the kids slept in the fort that separates the boy swing and the girl swing.

"The fort was fun, cold, and scary," she told me. "We watched two movies, and I got bit by a million mosquitoes, but I loved it! Can we sleep in it tonight, too?"

During treatment when our schedules got crazy, I brought Abigail to my yoga classes for my own practice. She was five and had mastered the concept of *quiet time* while I got *mommy time.*

She explained, "I remember I would play puzzles in the yoga room until it became time for savasana. Then I would lie on your belly and fall asleep. You would scratch my back. Sometimes I would get a mat and practice next to you. I remember the other people would smile at me. I felt shy when this happened."

School let out early on Fridays, and sometimes, if Michael and I couldn't juggle the schedule enough, I would bring the kids to the hospital during my radiation treatments. No flexibility in that schedule.

"One time, during radiation, I remember the nurses were sitting with me and teaching me how to draw good ghosts," Abigail continued. "Benjamin wasn't there. I remember the puzzles. I liked the puzzles. One had a sunset and a sky. I finished one by myself."

During the latter half of October, and with two weeks left in my radiation schedule, the kids had prepared their costumes and our house for Halloween. By now, hospital visitations were so thoroughly integrated into our routine that memories of a time when we didn't need to schedule it into our lives seemed long, long ago.

"I remember watching Mommy on the radiation table with red, green and blue lights everywhere around the room. I think they were coming from the machine. I thought they were lasers. It was a little scary," said Abigail.

I'm sure the theme of Halloween and my general appearance played a large role in their world of people becoming something that they're not. I wore my radiation costume.

"You were wearing a bandanna," Abigail told me, "And you had no hair on your face. It was weird. It was cuckoo to have both parents who were bald. I felt embarrassed at times. I wanted you both to have hair. It would make better sense for me."

We snuggled together on the couch in our living room prepared to read a book, and she curled against my body. Although we both knew that a *normal* looking mommy lived in our past and not in our present—yet the weight of her relief knowing that I could still BE her mommy, pressed heavily into my side. I held onto her, to maintain the strength that she required.

My brave daughter.

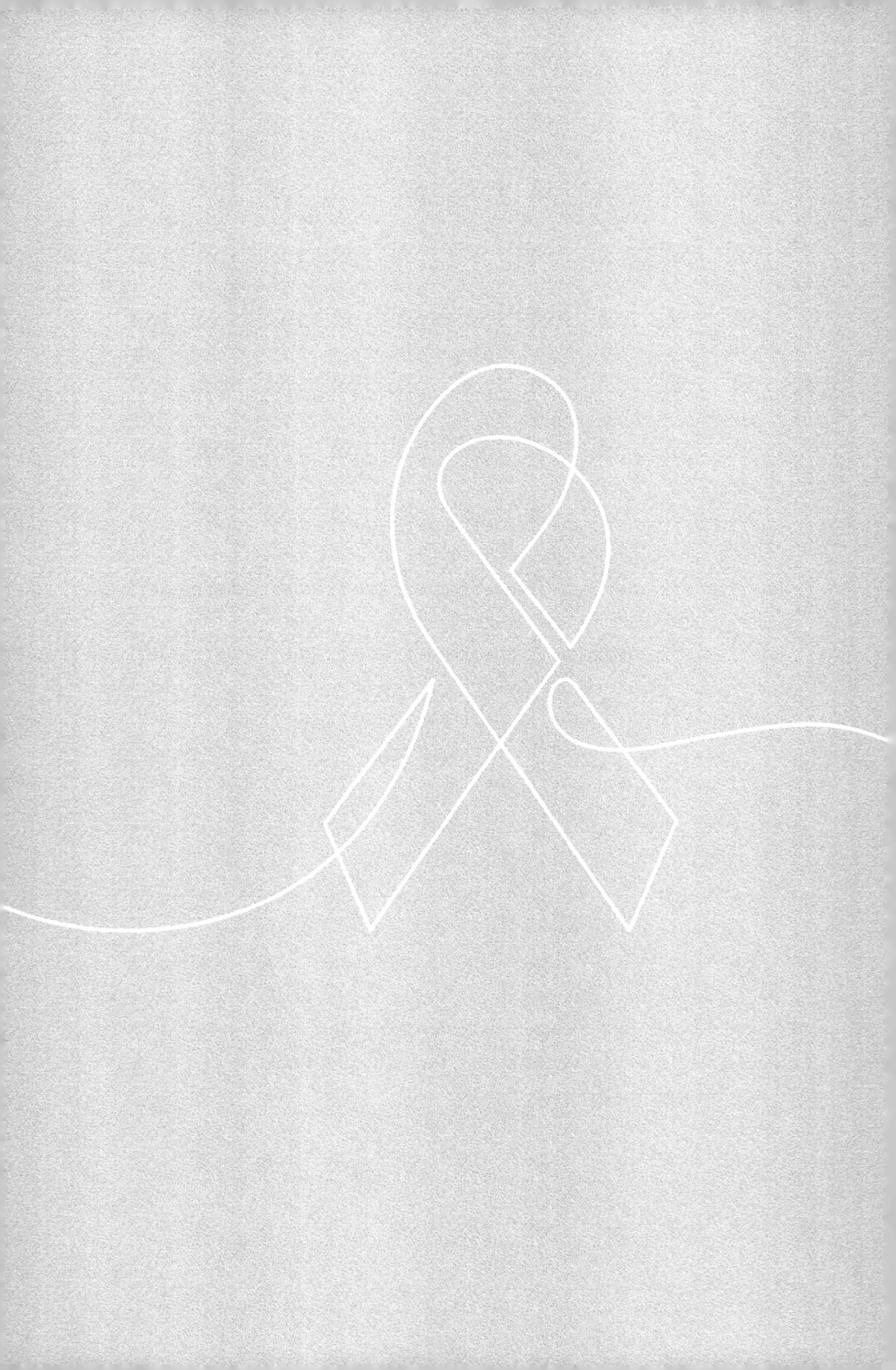

Mashed Potato Day

*If you can give your son or daughter
only one gift, let it be enthusiasm.*
—Bruce Barton

On a day that I had a bone scan scheduled, I was required to go in at 10:00 am and then again at 1:00 pm for the two-part test.

I had arranged for my children to have fun at a swimming pool with friends, but Abigail woke up on the wrong side of the bed and would have none of it. I explained to her that the alternative would be to follow me around all day—two doctors' appointments and one meeting.

"Kinda boring, Abigail," I warned.

She repeated over and over, "I just want to be with you today."

A big tear slid down her cheek. I backed down and acquiesced, "Okay," and I wiped it away.

It was the day after Christmas, and she was exhausted. Even playing with friends seemed like it would take too much effort.

The snow from the night before had piled up to the consistency of mashed potatoes.

Abigail liked that and stomped her feet all the way from the parking lot to the hospital entrance. "Stomp. Mash those potatoes, Mom! Stomp."

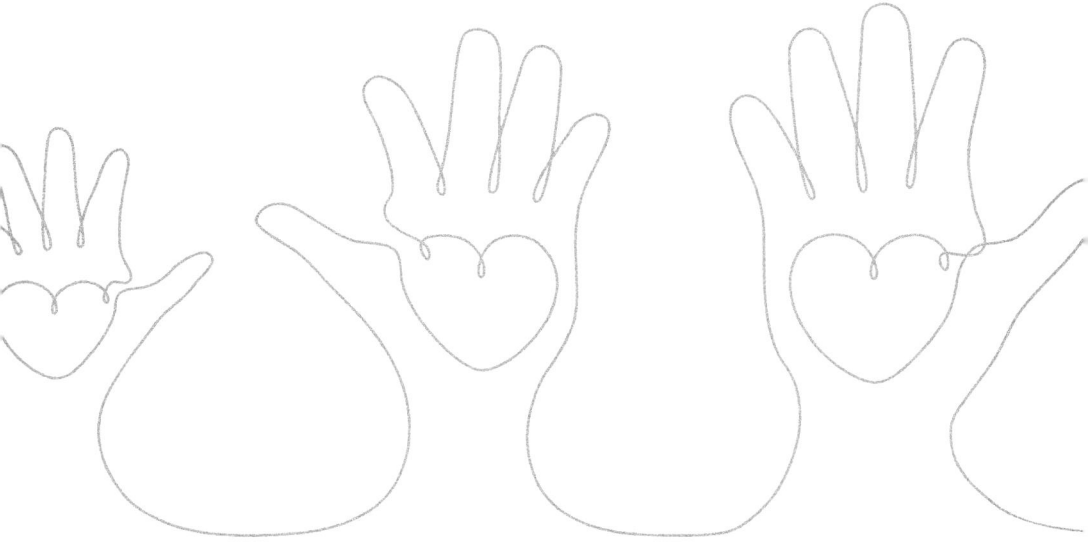

PART THREE
My Community

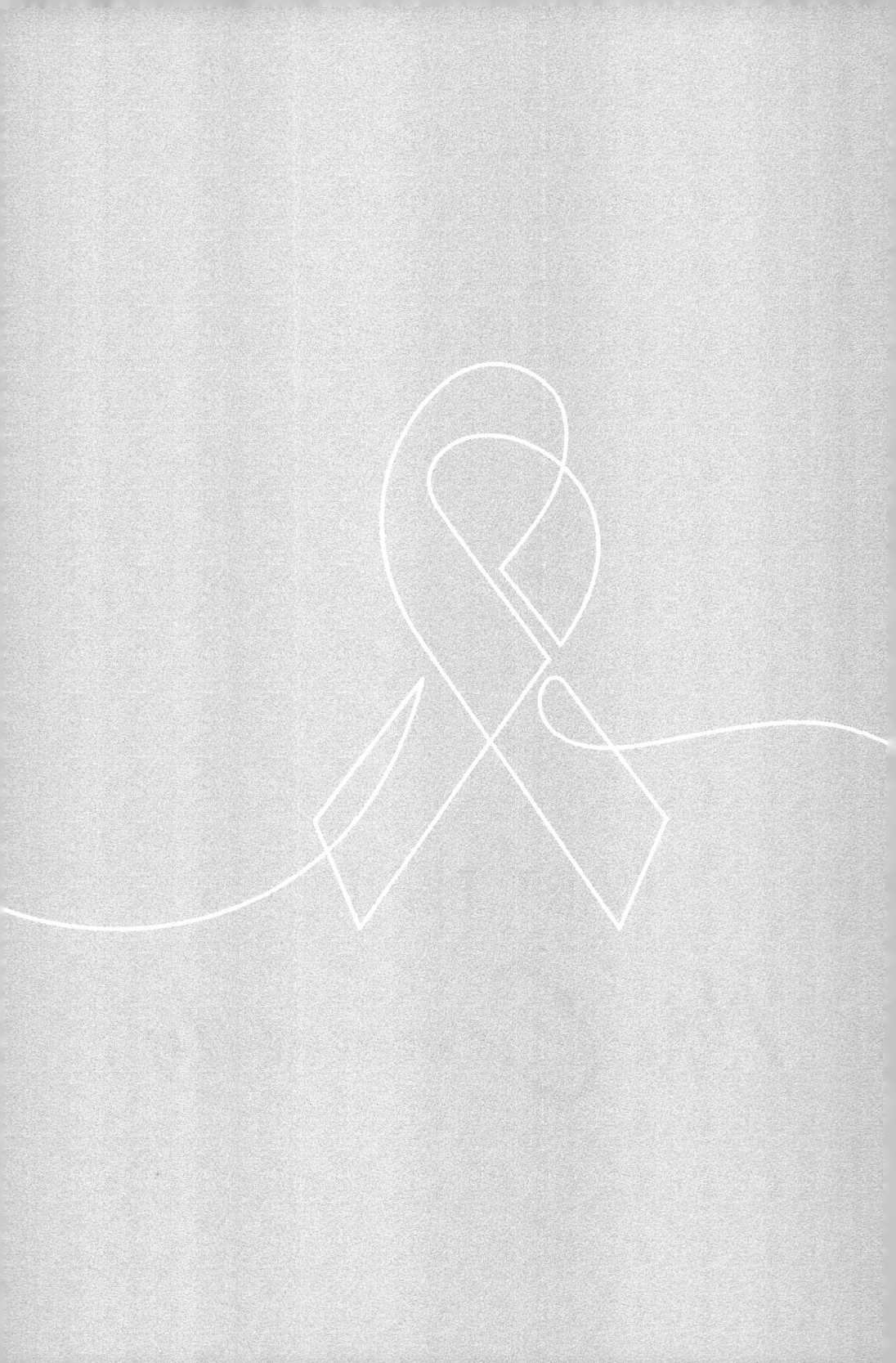

Firefighters

*"I will never allow personal feelings, nor danger to self,
deter me from my responsibilities as a firefighter"*

—Firefighter Code of Ethics

When your life takes a sudden turn and the unexpected lies before you, the simplest of questions can appear overwhelming, and relying on others for assistance becomes a temporary way of living.

It's foreign ground. Only trust in the guidance sustains you.

To understand a firefighter completely and not be one yourself means you're married to one or pretty darn close to one. Firefighters are a complicated breed. Their common features extend beyond state lines and even national borders. But the thing is—the very thing that drives you nuts about them—is also that thing that makes you love them.

Michael considers it an honor to be a firefighter, and I honor him in discovering and living his passion. He is great at what he does; yet he would never admit to anything more than being just one of the guys within this group.

I started anticipating the events of September 11, 2001, about six months before it happened, and about four years before cancer would hit our family.

Up until August, these premonitions came in the form of dreams. Then a terrible sadness started hitting me in the middle of the day, with no apparent reason. I would be driving and find myself needing to pull over because I couldn't see through my tears. The wave of emotion would last a few minutes, and then I could carry on with the rest of my day.

When the twin towers in New York fell, Benjamin was three and Abigail was one. I had slept in that morning, something I never did. I woke up when Michael came home, still in uniform from all-night duty.

He stuttered, "There has been a terrible accident. They think a small plane hit one of the twin towers in New York." His hands seemed to need a task. He actually signed *accident* and *plane.*

Later, the facts became clearer, the horror documented in every media format on earth. I found myself clinging to specific stories.

I want to know how the buildings were built! Why did the chiefs send those firefighters into those buildings? Planes hit those buildings! They can't put out those fires.

I was incensed—angry, and sad.

Although I know the code of firefighters, I was still infuriated that they followed it into such danger. I projected my own relationship with Michael onto their situation until I realized the true source of my fear. There was no separation between *us* and *them*. All firefighters believe in one thing, "To bring each other home safe to our families."

What happened in New York was felt across the world, but I witnessed it first-hand in my husband's anxious pacing. He was ready to go, waiting for the telephone call that would mobilize him.

That call never came, although some Salt Lake County firefighters were sent to New York. His job was to stay out and cover home base.

I finally received the answer about the architect and to my

demands for more information on the building's structure. It was aired on PBS about nine months later.

We were in Chicago, visiting friends and family. The fear of tall buildings coming under attack was still very fresh on everyone's mind. Chicago has the tallest building in the United States, and we were hearing about precautionary procedures and structural integrity—very different information than what we were used to getting as tourists on our earlier visits.

People there were not at ease.

When I heard the story about the "Six fire fighters from Ladder Company 6" and their guardian angel, Josephine, I was able to release my anger toward the fire chiefs who orchestrated the rescue efforts on that fateful day.

I read about the story first, then saw a TV interview with the firefighters and Josephine. I remember chuckling at their obvious discomfort with the interviewer's efforts to make them admit they were heroes.

Six men, each carrying over a hundred pounds of equipment, entered the building where everyone else was escaping from. They found Josephine, a sixty-year-old grandmother, inside the stairwell of the north tower. She had been on the seventy-third floor and had trudged down sixty stories before she sank down, exhausted. The six firefighters had reached the twenty-seventh floor, four levels past Josephine, when they heard the south tower fall. They turned to retreat and stopped where Josephine had slumped to the steps.

One of the firefighters hooked Josephine's arm over his shoulders while he put his arm around her waist to guide her down the stairs.

He encouraged her, "Josephine, your kids and your grandkids want you home today. We've got to keep moving!" The progress was extremely slow. The threat of the building collapsing loomed large.

On the fourth floor, Josephine gasped and stopped.

"That's it. I can't go anymore."

That's when the tower went down. Hearing the rumbling, like an approaching train running full force, the firefighter who had been guiding Josephine calmly told her, "Josephine, I'm going to place you in this doorway and shield you with my body."

He did. He said he could feel and hear the floors below them give way and the floors above them crushing down.

The only pocket that survived, walls intact, in the north tower of stairwell B was between the second and the fourth floor. After six hours, all six men from Ladder Company 6 and Josephine, were rescued.

Rescuing people is part of the job. Michael is a paramedic, too, and many of his calls are medical ones. When he rescued an unconscious six-year-old found hiding in a closet from a fire and was able to revive her, he considered that day to be a pretty good one, but he keeps it in perspective. That's what he does. It's his job.

When a fellow firefighter is in danger, his peers exert the same amount of effort to rescue him, but there is a subtle shift in perspective. Michael has often referred to the fire department as a group of men and women who are bound together by an unspoken oath.

If a firefighter is down, everyone bands together to lift him or her up. It's our job to bring everyone home safe to our families.

When Michael and I were going through our cancer marathon, this unspoken code went into effect immediately, much of it without our awareness. There are three-hundred and eighty firefighters in the department. Michael works closely with about fifty of them, but all of them heard the news. Over a four-month period twenty firefighters shaved their heads honoring their friend Michael, honoring him, honoring me.

"If one of us is bald, then we're all bald."

A friend told us about a firefighter who had the most adorable set of curls atop of his head. "They're magic," his wife would say. When everyone around him started shaving, he thought he should, at the very least, talk to his wife about it. Her reply was simple, "I love your curls, but you can shave them off for your friend."

About a week after the bald party, Michael was filling out paperwork at the station when one of his buddies walked up and handed him a check for five hundred dollars. Civil servants typically don't have large bank accounts. A lot of firefighters have the job as their passion but actually have to hold down a second job to pay the bills. Michael wasn't sure how to respond, but he understood it. "A fellow firefighter is down, and we need to lift him up."

There are three hundred million people in the United States and only one million firefighters (70% of them are volunteer), all of them rotating in shifts. When they're in sync, they can silently move together, matching motion to assist strangers, bringing them out of burning buildings, stabilizing them, preventing them from dying, sending them off in the ambulance, and turning to the next one. It's a dance, a movement, that occurs without speech because they know each other so very well. I've heard Michael say, "We may never have the opportunity to share a beer together or to shoot a game of pool, but we're all connected just the same, in this common space in time."

In 2006 we attended the annual firefighters' banquet. Two of the three platoons were in attendance, everyone in formal blues. These guys and gals never see each other all in one place unless there is a huge fire.

Michael is happy to see everyone. "It's like a reunion."

What I didn't expect was the attention that I received. From the administrative assistant to the chief and every rank in between. They were asking how I was doing.

My hair got lots of attention. "Look at all that hair!" and "I haven't seen you two since you were both bald!"

Time hadn't passed for many of these people, we were frozen in it. The evening was filled with hearty handshakes and belly laughs, but it was the connection—being able to close this particular chapter for the department. That was most memorable for me. I left feeling honored and blessed.

In the end, Michael's adventure was separate from mine. It included all of these people whom I will seldom see many I will never even meet. Hundreds of people hear the news, make inquiries, and continue to keep us in their prayers.

Once, when Michael and I were feeling brave, I asked him, "If we had to do it all again, could we?"

It was a difficult question for both of us, triggering way too many emotions.

He finally said to me, "If you have to cross over difficult waters, I will build the bridge."

I won't question it. I don't. It is just the thing that needs to be done. I would do that for you."

We sat close together, quiet for a long time. I finally said, "I don't want to go through this experience again, but I know I could, with you by my side."

Like the firefighters in stairwell B of the World Trade Center, remaining together to save one, before the world came roaring down. "I'm going to lay my body over you to shield you, to protect you."

Michael and I felt this protection, from the department, his platoon, and each other.

Tarot Reading

*Get your facts first, and then you can
distort them as much as you please.*

—Mark Twain

My friend Jules flew in from Sacramento. She brought all the things I miss about living in California. Peets Coffee and Tea, fine wines, and a broad spectrum of thinking.

When Jules shared her stories with me, I experienced the essence of her spirit—how I missed that. We have memories of the small home-town community that are often forgotten.

In addition to the beauty of the Utah landscape, the immediacy of access to the mountains is such a gift that it helps me stay sane. But what I love most about this state is the feeling of community and the people who practice the art of taking care of one another.

If I had not gotten sick, I may never have known about them.

The Native American community, the holistic community, the athletic community, the mountain community, and the spiritual community. I have benefited from all of them and continue to seek them out when I am feeling "two quarts low" as Michael would say. (The man's from Detroit, after all.)

When Jules comes to visit, we have a routine. We get pedicures, massages, eat at One World Café, buy good coffee, and get a tarot reading at the Golden Braid Bookstore.

Barbara is our tarot reader. She is from Australia and stands about four feet nine inches in heels. She has red hair and looks beautiful in the color pink. She often tells me stories of her grown sons and their animals. She rarely speaks without a smile on her face.

During Jules reading, she laughs through the whole thing. I spend time at the koi pond between the bookshelves, listen to my children share books with one another, and wish the day would not end.

It always startles me to feel such peace and contentment during this time. I breathe it in and remind myself that I can accomplish this myself, whenever I desire.

When it is my turn, Barbara asks me to shuffle the cards and cut them into three piles; the magic begins.

I've had several readings from Barbara and am fascinated that each time the same cards get turned over. And just like in the movie *Sleepless in Seattle* the phrase *It's Magic!* pops into my head.

This is my impression. But more so, this is what I *believe*.

This time, each card I turned over Barbara told me something new. Michael and I have each shared past lives together (this I knew), but each of us had died before we had the chance to live fully (this I did not know).

This life is the first time that we have been able to *fulfill our contract*—to not have our time together cut short. It's as if we have come back for each other as a couple, as parents, as individuals.

Barbara's words chime in my heart with assurance.

I thought about my asthmatic childhood and Michael's endurance in traveling across the country with only spare change in his pocket. I thought about doing the cancer adventure together. We kept conquering difficult times and coming out on top.

Her words explode inside me, singing the reasons for living my life. I've felt the pull toward retreating, hiding, or becoming small, but energy surged within me—encouraging me, and others, to build bridges, to grow, and to flourish.

I came here to live my life. I accepted the obstacles, but I'm limber and negotiated around them. I'm here with Michael, and we're raising our children, and I'm laughing with Jules.

This is a life worth living.

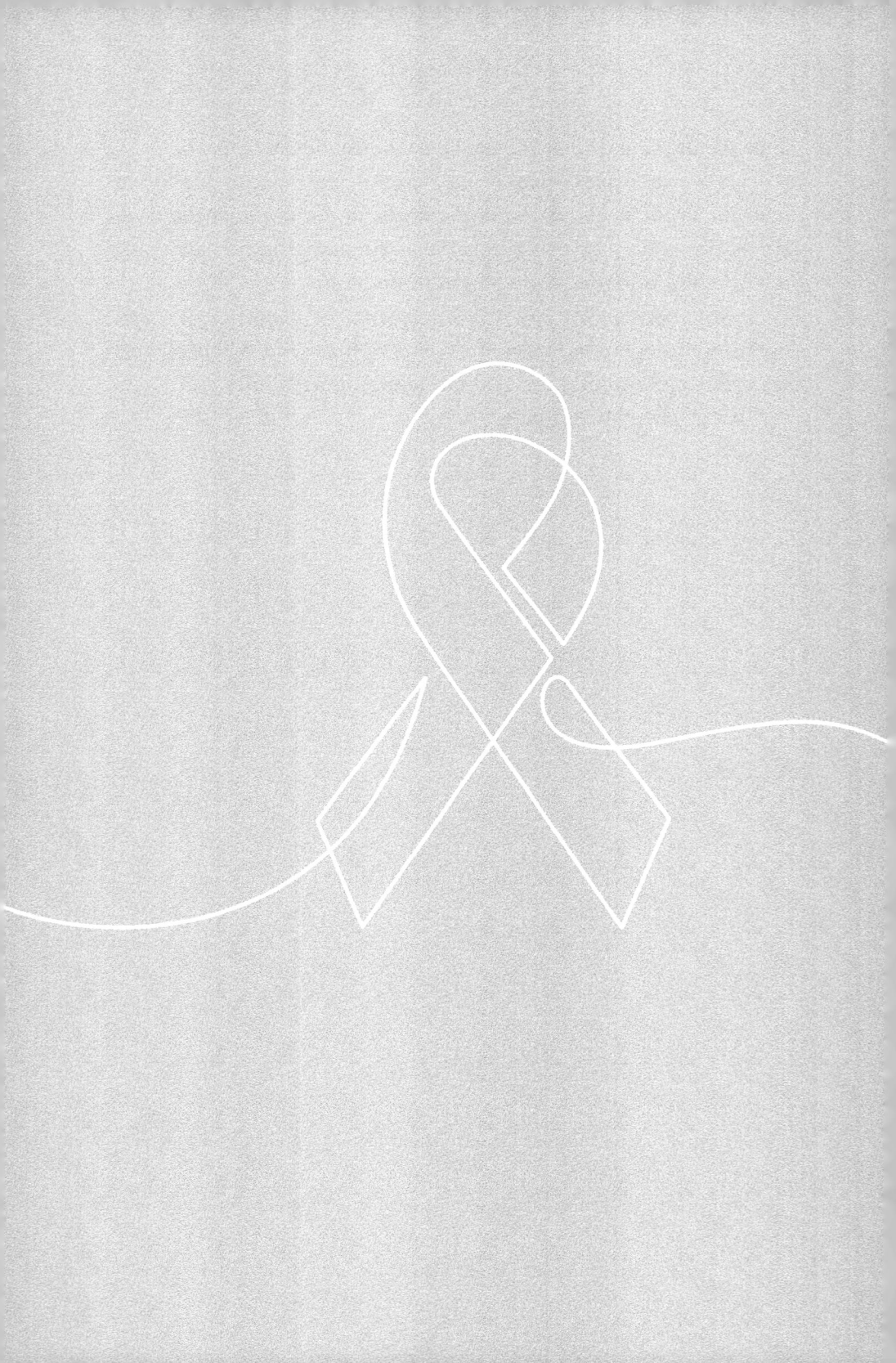

Rose

*Yesterday is history, tomorrow is a mystery,
today is a gift, which is why they call it a present*

—Master Oogway, (Kung Fu Panda)

If I could gather the people who kept us sane, hold them close, and press them near to my heart, who would they be?

It is true that I required the skills of my surgeons, oncologists, and their medical staffs to intervene and eradicate my tumor, lymph nodes, and ovaries. These trained professionals are a blessing.

It is true that our school communities cuddled us in the palms of their hands, providing a safe environment for Benjamin and Abigail to be children. Teachers and fellow co-opers, parent volunteers, lovingly intervened to eradicate fear. They truly were a blessing.

It is true that friends and family who lived far away provided support with love notes and airline tickets to eradicate tension.

They, too, are a blessing.

My immediate family never left my side. They made their own interventions of faith, will, and determination. They dismissed the question about the possibility of a full recovery.

They were *my* blessings.

The process of healing takes on many forms and what I have come to discover is much of the power behind healing has nothing to do with force, but rather with surrender.

Letting go—releasing.

Rose arrived as a gift from a friend but immediately embraced us, touching us with the same skills as my doctors, with the same love as our communities, with the kindness of our friends and family, and with the unquestionable faith of Michael and our children.

She is not one whom I seek out to find help from the outside. She is already within me.

Rose is a massage therapist, a clairvoyant, a healer. I have no interest in providing proof of her magic. "Is everything required to have an explanation?" No.

What I know is this: My lymph-swollen arm has returned to normal size. She has prepared my other arm, sclerosed veins and all, for future surgeries with no struggles to get the IV into my vein. She has helped dispel Michael of his own fear of my cancer. My children are calm in her presence.

She ratified my own thoughts and feelings. "In this life . . ." she paused, then finished the thought. "This life is for the living."

I cannot *reason* cancer. I cannot explain why it entered my life when it did, nor can I *explain* it. Why my energy level rose so rapidly following chemotherapy, and other patients did not. My doctors all witnessed my allergic reaction to a particular kind of chemo treatment, then saw the Pranayama technique. (Prama is life force and yama means control). So, Pranayama breathing stabilized and calmed my heart rate. I cannot reason any of this, nor the hundred more that happened for me.

On Saturday nights I taught Yoga Kids at the studio. I often closed the session with a book called, *Zen Shorts*. It's a children's book for ages six through ten, but really, it's for all of us.

In the story, a giant panda named Stillwater teaches three children three ancient Zen tales about acceptance, forgiveness, and generosity, relating them to events occurring in the lives of each of these children.

Like Stillwater, Rose gives reason to the chaos of cancer through stories and metaphors. She brings wisdom with each stroke of her healing touch as she works on our bodies, releasing our past from our present. In yoga, teachers often refer to unwanted emotions trapped within parts of our body that present themselves as pain or stiffness. As we open up our body gradually, we release these packed-in emotions, removing those obstacles.

In the warmth of Rose's massage room, she manipulates our muscles, to release tension. But it is more than merely physically relaxation. She holds our heads, enabling our minds to rest, giving us more than mere ease with our thoughts. We experience peace from within, for she cradled our hearts, assuring us that love is the ultimate healer, and that we can put down our burdens of yesterday.

No one had seen Rose for more than a week, but then she called. I knew that privacy and space were important to her, but I stopped by her house anyway. I dropped hand-written notes in her mailbox, expressing love and encouragement from the other side of her front door.

She told me that a long-time friend had committed suicide. She was just forty-six, but depression had left her too crippled to cope with life any longer. She hadn't been able to accept the many hands who reached out to help her.

Such news about any friend would be terrible, but for Rose, it was devastating. Her profession, actually, her mission and calling—is healing. But she couldn't save her friend from her own choices or heal her pain.

Rose was calling to thank me for my *love notes* and the reminder of what they represented She had a decision to make. Would she sink into the same darkness that had swallowed up her friend or turn toward love and light.

Rose chose love.

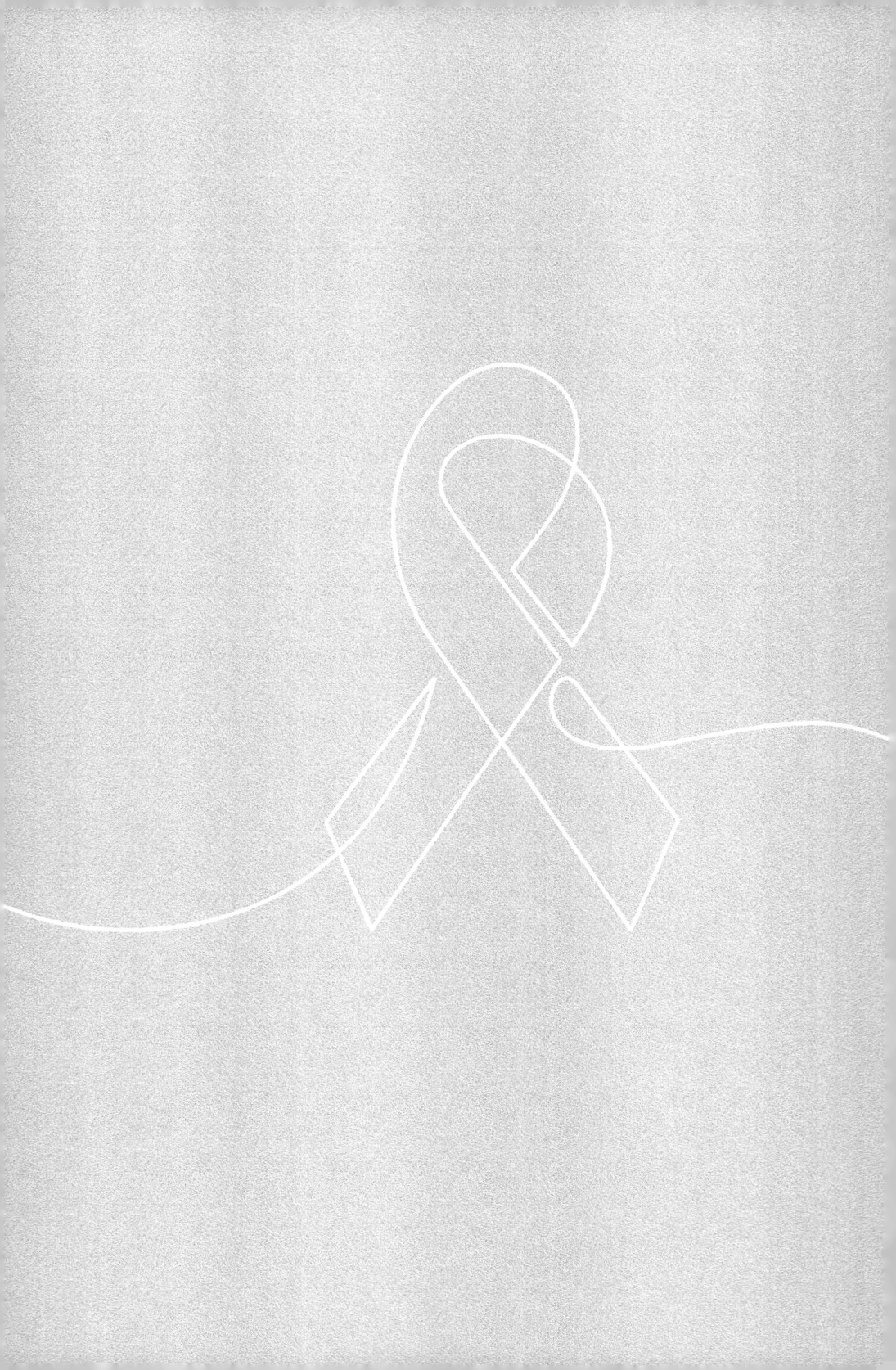

My "Y"

You gain strength, courage and confidence by every experience in which you really stop to look fear in the face.
—Eleanor Roosevelt

I practically grew up in the Armed Services YMCA. My father was a program director for a downtown port of Los Angeles/Long Beach YMCA from 1955 to 1975. My brothers and sisters and I spent our first ten Christmases at the YMCA.

My mother was nine months pregnant with my younger brother and found herself doing what she had been doing on Christmas morning since she married my father—making breakfast for 200 servicemen. While she was mixing biscuit dough, she suddenly felt a contraction and grabbed her belly.

My grandmother, my dad's mom, just looked at her and said, "Not now, Sue. We have biscuits to make."

My brother Christopher must have recognized the voice of authority as he waited to come into the world the very next day!

I often say, "I was raised by my parents and the YMCA." My local Y was the Los Altos branch. It was there that I became a camper, a counselor-in-training, a counselor, and eventually a camp director. I learned early that leadership and having fun can be synonymous. In those days, taking charge of twelve first graders at a Disneyland adventure or taking them all to the beach was simply another way of having fun.

The way the current laws are, in 2024, depending on the state, it's more complicated for organized day and resident camps. I do believe the fun factor still exists, if you're willing to make it happen.

As a child and teen, I spent time in resident camps. I attended Camp Oakes and Camp Whittle, located in the San Bernardino Mountains of southern California. Our adventures took us away from the city for an entire week into the mountains tall pines. We stayed in rustic cabins and shared a community bathrooms with four other cabins. With eight girls to a cabin, that was thirty-two girls!

The boys were on the other side of the meadow in similar circumstances. We had no heaters, and or electrical outlets.

It was true camping.

Designed into the overall YMCA camp experience were programs to help facilitate inner growth and development for the camper, counselor, and director.

There were specifically designed programs. Their symbols were a rag and a leather piece.

We folded a blue bandanna diagonally, making a triangular shaped *rag* that each camper wore around their neck. The three corners symbolized the body, mind, and spirit. The triangle shape symbolized the need to keep them all in balance.

The Ragger's program began almost ninety years ago when one camper had a physical disability that kept him from participating in the sport program. (The program celebrates its 110th birthday this summer—2024). Perhaps unaware of the significance of the gesture, his counselor awarded him the blue bandanna as recognition that he was participating with his enthusiasm and encouragement. As a result of this camper's natural intentions to support others with passion and without self-pity, the Ragger's program was born.

It has grown significantly adding seven colors of Rag. Each

color symbolizing a particular challenge in self-awareness and development.

The Leather program is for campers ages nine through eleven. This program was important to me. I'd set certain challenges for myself as a child, and the Leather focused that desire for achievement. The first Leather was also a triangle, again symbolizing body, mind, and spirit.

The Rag program was for ages twelve and up.

Utah's YMCA municipal building was fairly new to the state but the resident location, Camp Roger, has been in existence for over seventy-five years, established in 1948. Michael and I worked with camp director, Amy Henry. We introduced the ragger program to Camp Roger and were planning on sending our children to the camp. We considered this experience essential in contributing to their inner and outer growth process.

When I sit before my yoga students, all capable men and women, I consider it part of my responsibility to raise the awareness of those around me to remember the need for balance in body, mind, and spirit; equally weighted, equally strong.

Through certain poses we can *bring up stuff*, as my own teachers have explained to me. I am reminded that it is not our incapabilities that are causing our expressions of frustration or fear.

Rather, our ability to show these emotions demonstrates strength. Someone once told me, "It has often been thought that crying is a sign of weakness; but the fact of the matter is that it takes a lot of courage to shed a single tear."

Saying "I have cancer" aloud for the first time, and then *hearing* yourself say those words, can be terrifying. Those capable women who pride themselves on so many accomplishments suddenly find themselves at a loss emotionally when they experience that for the first time. hear themselves say these words aloud.

It is in their balancing of their capable mind, body, and spirit, that they meet the challenge and begin the healing process.

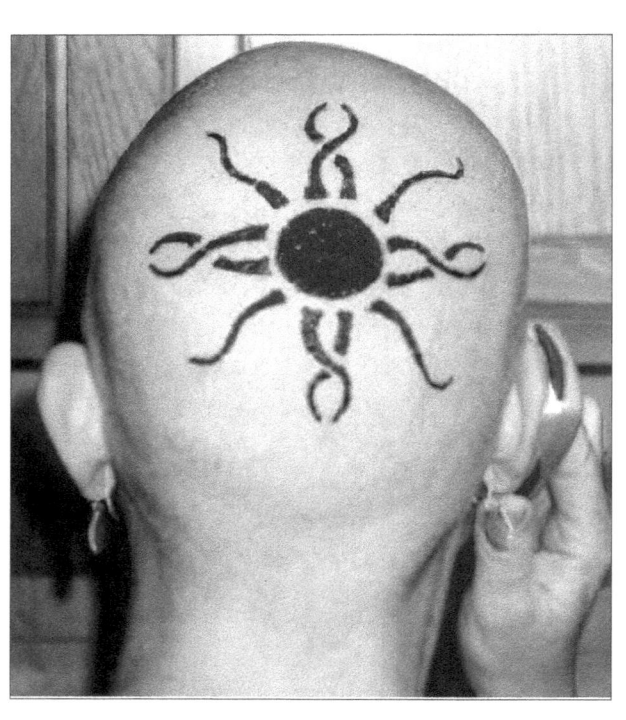

Moving Past the Fear

You are able to say to yourself, "I have lived through this horror. I can take the next thing that comes along." You must do the thing you think you cannot do

—Eleanor Roosevelt

"Does it ever go away?" Beverly asks. "When can I start to breathe again? I keep inhaling, but I haven't exhaled in two years. I need to exhale, but I'm afraid that, when and if I do, something else will release from me and I don't have that much left to release."

A student in my Quality Life Community yoga class, Beverly proclaims that her claim to fame is three mastectomies. She had one, then reconstruction. Cancer returned to the remaining authentic breast. She had it removed, as well as the reconstructed breast.

And now she is afraid. She keeps waiting for the next shoe to drop. She is one of the funniest women in the group and ironically, she hides her fear so well, so gallantly, so stylishly.

Most of us aren't that successful at deploying a survival technique so finely tuned to mask the emotion she doesn't like to feel—fear.

Facing fear must be done with consistency, confidence, and intensity. This is not easy, but it is the only way to knock it down. Otherwise, it wins.

Choose a mantra. *Release to be well*, or *Well body, well mind, well spirit*. Whatever works. The words are less important than the absolute emotion, the conviction, the assurance.

Praise your body for what it is doing. Phrase your messages to yourself without using *not* or *can't*.

I chose to stroke my right arm. "Thank you, arm, for draining lymph fluid into new channels and drainage ports."

I placed my hand over my heart. "Thank you for being strong and beating while I'm awake and while I sleep. Thank you for healing my wounds from the inside out."

The parts that are doing well, bathed in praise and gratitude, will help the parts that are out of balance. The energy within, practiced with consistency, confidence, and intensity, will make fear disappear.

Gratitude.

I'm a schoolteacher, and I praise students who are working with one another harmoniously, maintaining equanimity in the classroom, and hopefully, carrying that balance to the playground and beyond.

I know that, when I focus on their good behavior, it helps nurture balance within students who are not working together harmoniously. Positive behavior brings discordant behavior into harmony and alters emotions.

Disruptive students begin to feel differently about themselves. Soon the classroom is in balance. All I needed to do was set the process in motion with my positive words and attitudes, then not interfere with the momentum.

The process takes over and smooths away the knots.

So Now What?

God, give me guts.

— Eli Mygatt

Between the fall of 2005 and the spring of 2006, I became certified as a yoga instructor and started the A Quality Life Community class for cancer survivors, caregivers, and their loved ones. It was a free class offered at the studio where I trained.

Eventually, the class sustain itself through referrals, with very little advertisements.

My students often asked, "So now what do we do?"

These are common question. "Do we just wait and see? Do we pretend nothing really happened?"

The problem lies in an inescapable reality.

"I lost a year of my life."

I simply cannot ignore this, nor would I expect anyone else to. I cannot live as if I'm waiting in the sidelines of my life. That means I'd be waiting for my life to run out, and that is not me.

I suppose I was seeking the security of someone to tell me, "Your life is yours, now. Go live it."

What is it about my body and cells that differ from Michael's? Why did my cancer cells come out of dormancy and become activated? Did I live a stressful life? Did pregnancy trigger just the right chemical reaction to stimulate growth? Did I breast feed too long? Not long enough? Why did my cancer cells begin to grow?

And now I sit on the other end of the adventure wondering which way to move forward.

I've been repeatedly told, "You got the green light now hit the ground running. Do you allow yourself the time to sit to read a book?"

This is true; I've been running. I don't want to run out of steam, but I find too many things urgent, and I know I'm capable. The truth is too, that I have a pile of books on my bed stand. How long will they wait?

I'm moving forward to be still within myself.

Stillness is not death, it is listening. With yoga I practice my stillness. I'm working on bringing more of that into life. This is not to say that I will be stoic, or expressionless, or monotone.

It is to say, as John Muth writes in his children's book, *Three Questions*, to help explain 'Why we are here?'

When is the best time to do things?
Who is the most important one?
What is the right thing to do?

The most important are the people I am with. The right thing to do is to listen and respond to them. And now is the best time.

My children are in this answer. As they grow and develop, their complexities become, well, more complex. With each passing day, I am shown another layer of their thought patterns and emotional development. Each and every day, I learn more about their interests and curiosity. I find myself needing to stay abreast of these developments. Childhood is only ten minutes of our lifetime; I don't want to waste it rushing out the door to run to some event that only takes me away from them.

Cancer took away a year, but perhaps it gave me a perspective that I would not otherwise have. Would I have pursued my three questions? Would I have listened to my children's thoughts? Would I have taken the time to read for myself? Would I have taken the time to be still?

I am now moving forward. With this motion, I take with me this wisdom of stillness. It's not a particularly easy task.

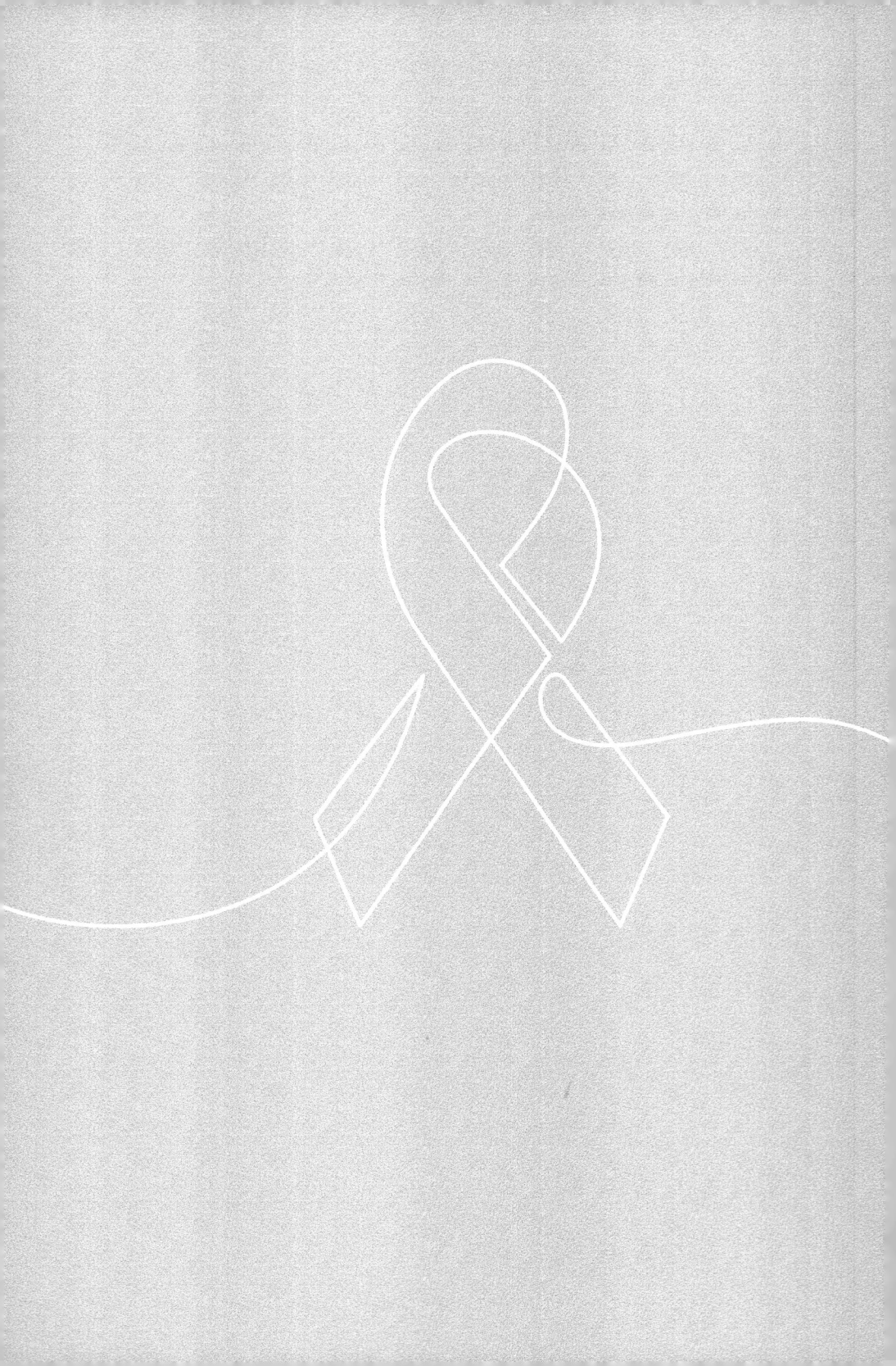

Remembering, Memorializing...

Life is either a daring adventure or nothing.
—Helen Keller

The only other time I met with my bandana buddy Kelly, was outside The Coffee Garden, just a week before she died, defeated by the combination of the two forces, cancer and chemotherapy.

Valentine's Day was approaching, and I brought her a heart-shaped cookie and her favorite tea from The Coffee Garden. She cried when she first saw me, then laughed when she saw the tea. If she couldn't meet me there, she knew I would bring her favorite tea to her.

Her body was now frail, she had difficulty raising her left arm. Her cancer had settled on the left side of her body. Even with the absence of eyebrows and eyelashes, her smile hadn't changed. We shared a warm conversation in a loving space of time. In the silent admission that our paths would soon separate. I stood in her kitchen with a full heart, mourning her absence that had not yet taken place. I remember looking into Kelly's eyes and seeing, for the first time, her own acceptance of where her path would take her.

This moment we shared, in the presence of her husband Joe, gave purpose to all the effort extended in our attempts to defend life. My relationship with her from that moment on would be memories recalled in the company of her widowed husband. She is someone I still grieve for today, yet I'm grateful for our yoga communities that brought us together.

A month after Kelly's passing, the yoga studio held a memorial service for her. An Irish woman raised in the *Show Me!* state of Missouri, Kelly was a woman not to contend with! *Show me!* was essentially what Kelly was asking of all of her doctors when they diagnosed her with Stage IV lung cancer. It came just one month after she and Joe relocated to Salt Lake City.

When she signed the multitude of legal documents involved in purchasing a home, she told her realtor, "Now I can take care of this nagging cough. I'm sure it's skeletal-muscular. I must have pulled something."

A week later, she was delivered the diagnosis that didn't fit into her life's plan. I can still hear her defiant *Show me!* challenge as she, Joe, and her doctors designed an attack against the killer in her lungs.

Ironically, Kelly's whole life was about being physically active. She had won the state championship in track and field with three teammates as a senior in high school in 1983. A dozen marathon medals hung in her house. Her garage housed a variety of outdoor gear, motor and pedal bikes. Joe and Kelly, whether together and separate, were about being active and outdoors. Whether they were riding bikes from the Pacific Coast to Missouri or traveling through Ireland the same way, she relished the adventure of the journey.

The yoga's studio owner taught the most advanced class; this is where I met Kelly. We both wore bandannas and complained about the heat while we powered through our chaturangas, but we eventually adjusted to the heat to meet the challenge of the class.

We knew it was the added combination of chemo-induced menopause and the occasional hot flash that added to the heat of the studio that brought on our whining.

We would begin the class with greetings and end it by adjourning to the Coffee Garden for a latté and a green tea.

Relief.

Kelly's adventure lasted two years, which is absolutely phenomenal for Stage IV lung cancer. Near the end of her life, Kelly worked with an intuitive massage therapist who helped her with her passing. She called hospice and planned out her last days. She asked Joe to take her to the treadmill at the local gym for one last run/walk.

She died three days later—the day after Valentine's Day.

We held her memorial at the yoga studio, honoring her strength that far exceeded her physical body. Joe wrote a blog describing her accomplishments, her love for animals and kind people, how she earned two master's degrees in physiology working with cardiac patients of all ages. He summarized, "She always kept the focus on how she could use her own abilities to help others."

I helped Joe clean up after the memorial. At one point, I held a shadow box filled with medals and the photo of Kelly with her high school mates holding up the state championship plaque, all of them grinning from ear to ear. A set of identical twins "bookended" Kelly and the other girl in the center holding the plaque.

As we were both admiring the photo and the half dozen medals, Joe pointed to the woman standing next to Kelly.

"She just gave me a call."

The blog Joe had posted had connected and reconnected people from throughout Kelly's lifetime, both preceding and during their eight-year marriage.

"Her name is Julie. She was wondering if Kelly had told me the story behind this picture."

I look at him quizzically. "I had only heard that Kelly was extremely proud of this moment and that the twins were very fast."

He looked down at the photo again. "Julie told me that the first runner, one of the twins, had trouble getting her pace and made a slow start. By the time, the baton reached Kelly—she was second—her team was in seventh place. Once she got the baton, she took off! By the time she passed it to Julie, who was third, her team was one yard behind the first-place team. Only one yard!"

Tears pooled in his eyes when he looked at me. "Julie told me that it was Kelly's run that let them win the championship that day." He laughed softly, "She hated to be passed up by anyone."

We had held Kelly's memorial just days after Elizabeth Edwards, the wife of vice president nominee John Edwards during the in the 2004 campaign, announced that her breast cancer had returned. Elizabeth broke a rib while moving a trunk, and they found her cancer had metastasized to her bone. She and John considered the broken rib fortunate, since early discovery could mean that they had more time to make an action plan.

"Always finding a silver lining," Ms. Edwards added.

We shared the news at my yoga class for cancer survivors, her story reverberating like a gong through us. Fear, especially fear of cancer's return, is probably the biggest hurdle to jump.

"When I'm done with treatment, I want to be done with cancer," is practically a mantra, sometimes phrased in defiance, sometimes as hope, sometimes a prayer.

In 2005, when I was given my own diagnosis, my mother wrote a letter to Elizabeth Edwards. Somewhat to our surprise, Elizabeth responded with a hand-written letter to my mom, a testament to her character, especially during these days of email and text-messaging. In the letter she wrote about my mother's own recovery from breast cancer, then offered comforting words about the discovery of my own. The letter was a page long, written during Elizabeth's personal cancer adventure.

When my mom passed the letter onto me, her intention was clear; to share the wisdom it contained; strength. One of the women in my A Quality Life Community class had read Elizabeth Edwards's book *Moving from Grace*. She was moved by Elizabeth's ability to eloquently express her feelings, including the ever-present and sometimes overpowering fear and then, almost within the same sentence, use these same words to set fear aside, allowing space for healing.

Elizabeth Edwards has given birth to four children, spread across a whole decade. She lost a child when he approached adulthood. She has endured the limelight as the spouse of a popular senator and presidential candidate—twice!—as well as the sullying sensationalism of her husband's affair push all the other news off the front page.

Her personal challenges exist, but do they dominate her life? Her lifestyle is beyond busy, her expectations high. I found myself in awe at her kindness when I took the letter from my mother. We shared womanhood and its terrible fragility; I marveled at her assertion of optimism.

Does it seem so impossible that the power of optimism, love, and community would generate healthy cells, enabling the healing process to take place?

"Show me!" once glistened in the eyes of Kelly, my bandanna buddy. Elizabeth's letter encouraged my mother and me to draw from internal strength, to use what is already inside each of us. "Write!" I quietly utter, seeking the truth of the *power within* for surviving.

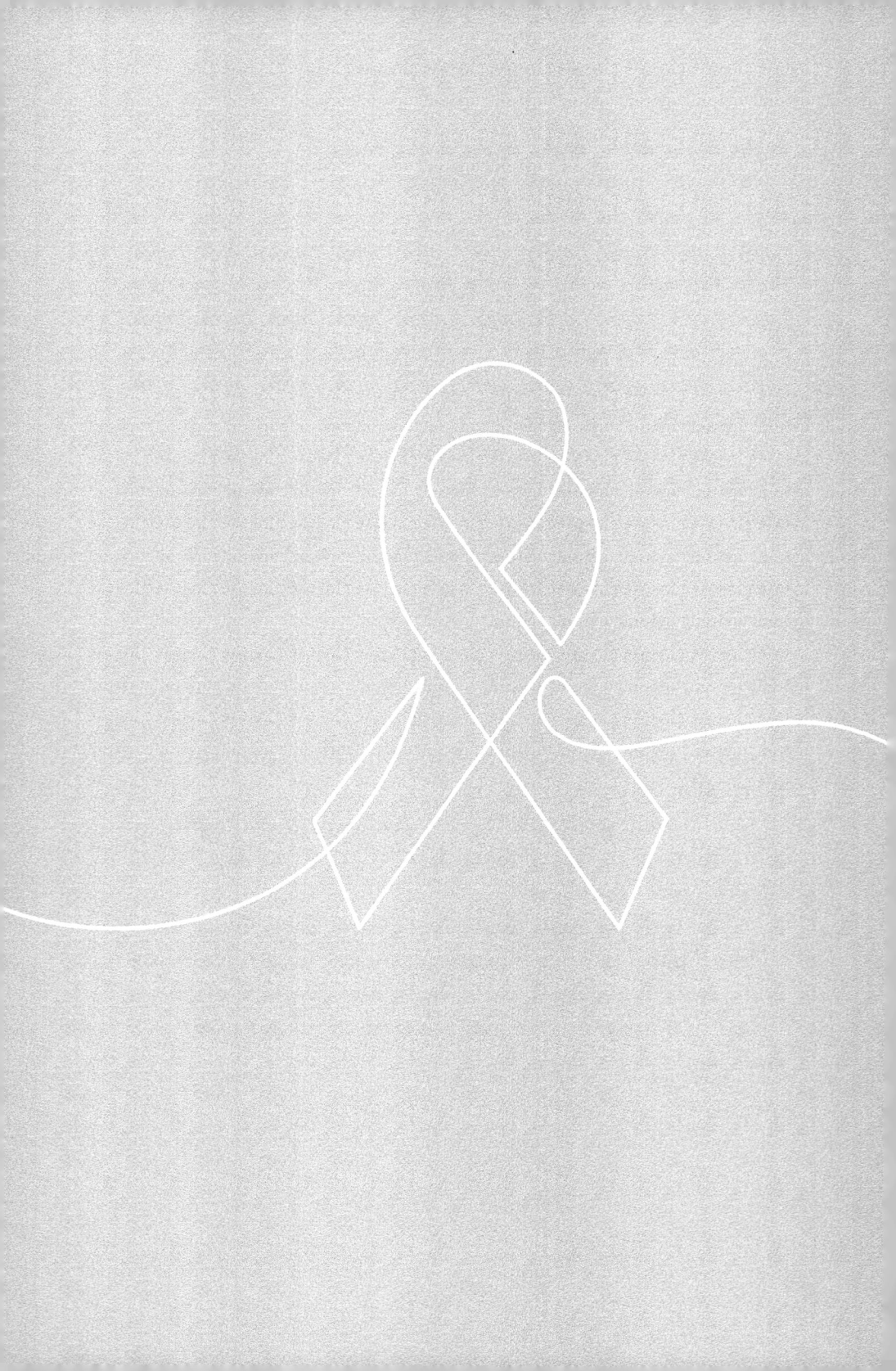

Beyond the Shadow of Doubt

That's the way things come clear. All of a sudden.
And then you realize how obvious they've been all along.
—Madeleine L'Engle

I volunteered once a week for Coming Home Hospice in San Francisco's Castro District. This hospice served a population consisting primarily of young men in advanced stages of AIDS. It was 1987, and many of the remedies used today were not available then.

Animal-assisted therapists were allowed to enter such facilities, thanks to the Society for the Prevention of Cruelty to Animals that trained dogs and owners. My first dog, Gwen, the cutest Springer Spaniel ever, had been certified.

When we entered the building, Gwen would go her route and I would go mine, individually visiting the people on our separate rounds. At this stage of living, some residents don't want greetings from people, so a dog was perfect.

Hospice care, or palliative care, is for the very end of life. I was assigned to Will and his mother.

"He's fighting," the nurses told me.

I was confused. "Fighting?"

"Yes. He is fighting death right now. He's working through something, so he is not letting go."

The nurses gently explained once in a while, this happened. Will and I were neighbors when I lived in the Castro District. He owned an antique store, and I remembered him being very tall.

Our last conversation was when we had a cup of coffee together at the corner café while our clothes were in the wash at the neighborhood Laundromat. When I saw Will in his bed he couldn't speak, and his mother only wept. They had been estranged for a long time.

When the Coming Home staff called her, she didn't know her son was HIV positive, that he had AIDS; that he was dying.

I noticed that his *fighting* and his mother's arrival appeared to share the same time frame. My first job was to help the nurses turn him and bathe him so that he didn't develop bed sores. My second job was to comfort his mother. She spent a lot of time wiping his eyes and then wiping her own.

Although my involvement with Coming Home Hospice provided me with evidence of the power behind the human spirit, I had not discovered the application of this power as it transformed itself into a healing remedy until I had experienced cancer myself and then, later, witnessed it in other people.

For me:

"My tumor shrank when I meditated and visualized it smaller."

"My depression disappeared when I began holding my body in inverted yoga poses."

"My arthritis left when I began a Pranayama practice."

Virginia Veach, of the Ting-Sha Institute in the bay area explains, "It's in these moments of silence or relaxation that healing occurs. Yoga, meditation, and relaxation are ways to quiet our minds. Relaxation is a state of openness and readiness. It is neither tension nor flaccidity, but availability for movement."

Often time, however, our lessons do not come in the form

of science or double-blind studies demonstrating beyond the shadow of a doubt, that yoga works. They are just stories from real people with real experiences. Somehow, yoga helps to release whatever they were holding onto that was defining their state of being. After breathing exercises, a tingling sensation is felt in the chest and then throughout the body.

"Prana," Virginia clarified. "Life energy—healing energy"

After class one evening, I met Arnold. His son Damian had lived with brain tumors from age eleven to his current age, twenty-eight. His sister, Nicki, took the A Quality Life Community class to learn how to alleviate some of Damian's pain. Damian's large tumors were successfully removed when he was twenty-three, but he still lived with three smaller ones monitored by his doctors.

The last surgery created a clot six inches long that caused a debilitating stroke. His body is now stiff and lethargic, his energy low. Leaving the house is a struggle against depression and constant fatigue. Nicki and Arnold both want to help but aren't sure how.

Meditation helped before, and after the first surgery, so they were willing to try it again. Arnold and Damian would meditate together, visualizing the tumor shrinking, being eaten away by little Pac Man munchers who thrive on tumors. They visualized white healing light, using tapes and books to help guide them through this process. It helped soothe their anxiety and made them both feel more confident. Each practice left them in a general state of well-being.

When the surgeon removed Damian's second tumor, he discovered that it had shrunk since Damian's last MRI, pulling away from the brain tissue. The surgeon could remove it in its entirety, simply lifting it out. When he walked out to report on the surgery to Damian's parents, he actually started by saying, "You're not going to believe this, but…" He ended with, "Next month we're hosting an international conference on brain tumors and Damian's case is going to be our featured presentation."

The meditation had worked.

Sometimes, it is the combination and cooperation of the two worlds—the two medicines—that help to heal the heart and the mind of the whole person. We often forget this but are reminded when we revisit the breath, the mind and the body.

I spent five hours with Will and his weeping mother at Coming Home Hospice, then at 11:00 pm, Gwen and I left. Within the hour, he died. He had released himself from whatever he was fighting against. One of the nurses called me that night.

"Amy, he was peaceful looking, content with the decision he made."

"What about his mother?" I asked. "Was she there? Did you call her?"

"Honey, she stopped crying. Apparently, she stopped fighting too, and that's when he began to look peaceful."

Wordlessly but communicating by the spirit, these two people were able to make amends, crossing the gulf of whatever was keeping them apart. In the end, they met on common ground, and both let go.

Amazing Stories

History provides abundant examples of people whose greatest gift was redeeming, inspiring, liberating, and nurturing the gifts of others.

—Sonya Rudikoff

I ran the *Race for the Cure* with ten-year-old Benjamin in the spring of 2008. *Race for the Cure* in Salt Lake City is held around Mother's Day, which just happens to occur near my birthday. Three years ago, the days made a parade.

Friday, May 6th, my forty-fourth birthday, Saturday, May 7th *Race for the Cure*, and Sunday, May 8th, Mother's Day! That was the year of diagnosis and discovery. I used to think of *discovery* as the tumor. Now I believe that *discovery* is my new way of being.

I saw a young woman at the *Race for the Cure* in the survivors' tent retrieving her gear for the first time; hat, T-shirt, bag of goodies, and her first pink ribbon. Lots and lots of people to cheer her on. She had to still be in her twenties. At first glance I saw her bright face, youth, courage, and a willingness to keep moving forward. She wore a broad-brimmed hat and her *Race for the Cure* shirt.

I approached her with the desire to give to her what all those people gave to me when I needed encouragement. As she turned toward me I discovered her healthy pregnant belly. She was standing the way pregnant women do, massaging her belly one hand and supporting her back with the other. She was *racing* for two this day, making her *survival* even more urgent.

I touched her shoulder. When she glanced at me, tears clogged my throat. I wanted to scream encouragement but only managed to choke out, "You're doing great!"

She looked back at me, her eyes aglow with her power and youth. "Thanks," she swallowed hard. "Thanks a lot."

Then the chaos of the day moved us apart. I probably won't ever see her again, but I will never forget her. By her mere presence, she seemed to say,

Yes, I'm young. I'm a cancer survivor. I have the whole world ahead of me. Yes, I am pregnant with this amazing child and isn't it fantastic? And by the way, I'm bald due to toxic treatments to counteract cancer that I'm beating. I'm thriving.

Her image stayed with me. Her body may be compromised in ways that we cannot see. She may never be able to breastfeed her baby or have days when she is too sick to even hold her baby. She may be frightened. But the power of creating life supersedes life being broken down. Holes eroded by fear are filled up and planted with blooming flowers of love.

She's bald, but hey! so are newborns. Together, they begin a new life together.

The Work Behind the Work

Without courage, we cannot practice any other virtue with consistency. We can't be kind, true, merciful, generous, or honest."
—Maya Angelou

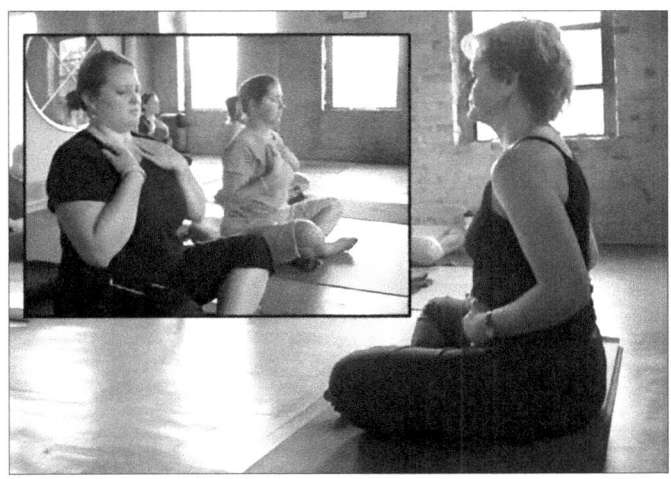

Before practicing Anusara yoga, our teacher will often set a *heart theme* or an *intention* for the practice of that particular day.

Our work on the mat most assuredly settles our minds, but what our work on the mat accomplishes also translates into work performed off the mat as well. Salkalpa, is the Sanskrit word for our intention and is likened to planting a seed—the work behind the work.

An analogy that I think best describes this practice is that of the farmer. At first, the physical labor—work of the farmer, may be tilling the soil and planting the seeds. The farmer knows this type of work so there is ease in his routine. With intelligence and forethought, he has mixed his soil with organic material, bringing it to the right temperature, and setting the ideal foundation for a seed to send down its roots, then send up shoots toward the sun. This is the work behind the work, establishing the perfect environment for his crops, which will then go on to feed a community. With the completion of the harvest, the cycle begins again with the next spring's preparation and planting.

In my yoga practice, I get my body to feel that it's not work—in other words, to find the ease within each pose to align my body so that works with me, not against itself. Yoga helps me become mindful, assisting me in placing my body, mind and spirit in a consciousness that allows me to do something about my intentions. Western civilization has the tradition of *powering* through the process, forcing an outcome to occur whether it be the intention or not. From the farmer's perspective, this would be similar to planting a bean seed but insisting on seeing a watermelon pop out of the ground.

Shashumna is the process of removing the kinks from our line of breathing. When we breathe with efficiency and without effort, from top to bottom and then back again, we find ourselves moving prana—life force—through our body. Heating our body, nurturing our body, allowing the energy from within to be extended and exerted outside our body, to the community. When this happens, we allow ourselves to get out of the way of the true work behind our intention. We find ourselves planting a bean and being perfectly content when a bean plant rises up from the ground.

Counting Taxis

One cannot divine nor forecast the conditions that will make happiness; one only stumbles upon them by chance, in a lucky hour, at the worlds end somewhere, and holds fast to the days, as to fortune or fame.

— Willa Cather

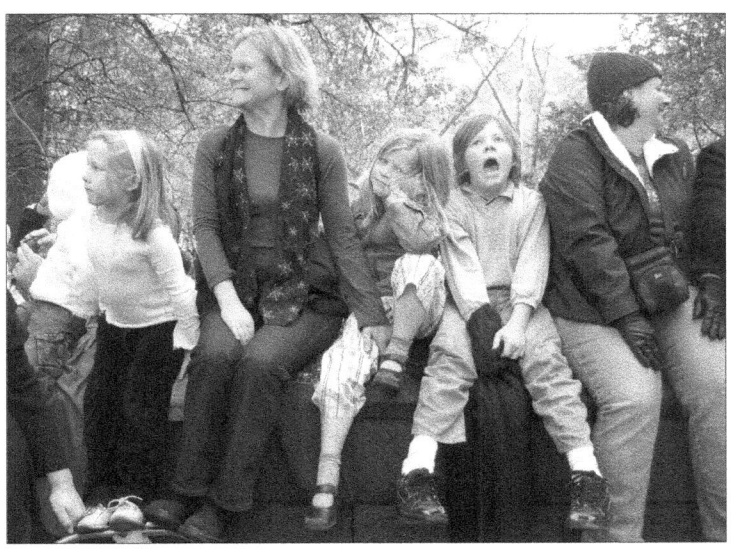

In November of 2007, two years since completing my treatment, our family flew to New York City during the Thanksgiving holiday so we could see the Macy's Thanksgiving Day Parade.

Cathy Simpson, a friend from my YMCA camp days, had lovingly found us a place to stay within walking distance of Central Park, so we could create a memory with our kids.

We had grand plans. We watched *Miracle on 34th Street* before we boarded the plane. A month prior to our trip, we watched *Sleepless in Seattle*. This video is a *must see* before our wedding anniversary. Don't ask me why. It just gets me in the mood for the season. That year Benjamin and Abigail watched it with us for the first time.

They were fascinated with the Empire State Building. "The building had a red light on it, and a red heart." Abigail loved this part so entirely that she drew the scene in her sketch book—our seven-year-old artist. So, I added up all of our frequent flier points, made about four hours of phone calls, and voila! We were on a plane to New York City.

This is my family's favorite time of the year. We love the fall. Michael and I were married in the fall. The season calls out to me, and I love the colors. It seems to say, "I'm yearning to be reborn and begin again, but for now, I'm tired and I need to rest."

Awaiting change myself, I correlate this response with my job as a teacher. I work with my students on topics that challenge their minds and their maturity. By springtime, I can already notice their change, their growth.

In the beginning of the year, our classroom *mantras* were *Be Aware of Your Surroundings* and *Raise Your Awareness*.

One student had such difficulty in adjusting to her body's growth spurt she would knock over computers simply crossing from one side of the classroom to the next. By spring, she was demonstrating leadership skills, assisting me in guiding the class rather than overpowering it.

In my own children, I find this inward growth more difficult to spot as I am with them all of the time. It is when I am away from them that I notice change. Lately, I find myself not wanting to be away from them, so I heavily rely on other people—their teachers and other parents—to give me hints about their growth. I am grateful for their feedback.

In autumn, I discover that I turn inward as well. As daylight savings time ends and darkness fills the night sky, I find myself heading home earlier and earlier. I cuddle in bed with nighttime stories with our children or snuggle in a comfy chair with my own books. I celebrate by letting those around me, my family, know that they are loved.

Fall, leading into winter, also offers a time for growth within our bodies from the inside out. It is my belief that our body tracks and mirrors the guidelines that nature lays out all around us.

New York is too crowded, and its residents know it. But the thing is, people who live there love it. They love speaking their mind. They love the frenetic motion. I spent one entire day traveling from one point to another in a crowd. It could have even been the same crowd. It was hard to tell. So many people.

I was meeting a friend in another part of town; and from the moment I left the apartment building until the moment I walked into his yoga studio, I was surrounded by a dense crowd.

There was, of course, peace within his studio, a nice reprieve; but we were hungry and needed to venture outside to *the crowd* once again. The restaurant was, of course, crowded. Service was slow. Impatience rose in waves from everyone around.

People seemed oblivious to what seemed obvious to me. Our minds and bodies don't do well with this much compacting. No one can be heard. It's hard to listen. The cell phone in my front pocket was set on high with an obnoxious ring/vibration, and I still couldn't hear Michael call me. This much sound impacts the spirit in a way that, I'm fairly sure, can only tear it down.

So, what draws seven million people to it? Opportunity and magic.

There is something to say about living in close proximity to other people for long periods of time. Does more isolation occur as a result of the physical closeness? I saw iPod earbuds in everyone's ears. I saw text messaging occurring non-stop with Blackberries in every location. I saw continuous and universal lack of eye contact. This behavior is considered common and predictable, while the less frequented emotion of a smile receives the most notice. It is the most unusual.

I returned from my friend's studio exhausted. I needed to take a walk, and the city had closed off has the road to cars on the inside of, Central Park. So, the space was even more open and the space even more quiet. I relished the moment. I walked briskly. It's cold enough that I need to keep moving or I'll freeze. The air is filled with memories of the fall. The people who share in my walk are spaced farther apart than my earlier experiences with them. They seem happier and more willing to exchange a glance. I breathe in and out and remind myself that I am here to participate in my rebirthing.

The next day my family and I are traveling across town in the underground subway. My son hears the subway conductor announce that our next stop is 34th Street.

"Mom! Miracle on 34th Street! This is the place."

Up to this moment, we were just another family on the subway. We had not made eye contact with the woman across from us. We hadn't smiled. We hadn't exchanged *Happy Thanksgiving* greetings.

But she smiled as she heard my son cry out in delight. Maybe she smiled at the thought that such magic still existed for a ten-year-old boy. I returned her smile, and we made a connection for that brief moment.

We confirmed my son's proclamation, "Yes, honey, this is the place. We'll visit Santa at Macy's and see what he has to say about this holiday."

Counting Taxis

Benjamin and Abigail were bouncing with excitement. All in all, this was a good moment.

When we got back to the apartment, Benjamin counted taxis from the front window. We looked down on the city in all of its New York glory. Lincoln Center would be lighting its Christmas tree on Monday. The ballet would be performing, and singers from the Met. We can enjoy it all from our living room window. It's absolutely magical.

As Benjamin counts the endless stream of taxis that dominate the streets, Michael doesn't have the heart to tell him that they are probably the same twenty taxis that just keep rounding the block. Nope. To Benjamin, this is a new sight to see. A new experience to feel. New sounds. We were ten floors up but could still hear the rain when it falls. We're absorbing the experience one minute at a time, not wanting to miss a single fragment.

Abigail notices that the snowflakes change colors with music. A new display across the street plays Christmas music, and the snowflake light fixtures respond with colors that dance in unison to the music. Together, they display Christmas to the eyes of a seven-year-old. But to be honest, Michael and I were captured by the magic as well.

We visited St. Paul's Church across the street. It used to tower above the street one hundred and fifty years ago. Now, high rises tower over it are on either side. Next we visited two-hundred-year-old St. Patrick's Cathedral. Finally, the Trinity Church near the Twin Towers site. Alexander Hamilton is buried there.

All of these ancient churches are huge yet dwarfed by the buildings that now surround them.

I can't help thinking, *They have survived for centuries. We are made small by their determination to persevere. People are drawn to these churches, these places of worship, of hope, and faith. Could it be that these buildings still exist because they understand the meaning of endurance?*

The next day is filled with the adventure at the Natural History Museum. This is a place especially for children, but it also provides us all with a message of the future. In the powers-of-ten display, the exhibit duplicates the event (or item) times ten toward the positive, then toward the negative, shrinking the event (or item) times ten. Each time, I'm drawn toward this side of the powers of ten, things made smaller. It is the cellular feature that fascinates me. It is the thing within me. Whatever it is that is biologically controlled, whether it operates on a cellular level or not, it is the thing that we cannot quite see that I am convinced attempts to run my body, challenges my body, perpetuates my body.

Each one of us has been affected by this town. With Michael, our firefighter and paramedic, we make a pilgrimage to visit the site where the Twin Towers stood. For Michael, this is a significant moment. It commemorated part of who he represented both as a man and as a professional. For the first time, the city's noise did not surround us. Silence replaced the sound. Without conversation, people walked the path and read the plans to build again—a design for hope, a representation that those who are not among us are still alive within us.

We lost a friend that fateful day, September 11, 2001. Christopher Newton left behind a wife and young children. His father hasn't been the same since. Outlining a plan for hope cannot be designed in haste. For this site, the plan is complicated and multilayered.

Carefully and with community support, such a plan is underway, fostering the healing process. Our last stop on this pilgrimage was Firehouse 10, a platoon that lost six members that day. A relatively small firehouse, it stands directly across the street from the site, on Liberty Street. They have saved the street sign and encased it in a frame. It is bent and crushed but the shape represents a wave, like a flag, rather than simply a bent-up piece of metal. There are symbols of loss everywhere in front of their station. The crowds linger here as much as they do on the site. It had been six years, and I can only imagine how the current crew of firefighters manage the crowd of people who visit their station. How can they deal with the overwhelming emotions and inquiry, the need for connection by the many onlookers? It is as if these firefighters have become celebrities without requesting it, working in a firehouse forever connected with this historical tragedy.

We came on a slow day. It was raining, and Michael was hesitant to knock. Earlier that day, we had asked a police officer if it would it be an imposition.

He assured Michael that, if he identified himself, he would be welcomed. It is a tradition among many firefighters to trade T-shirts with their city's emblem. When Michael and I took the kids to the Blue Mountains, outside Sydney, Australia, we met up with some firefighters who worked out of a small firehouse. During the ritual of trading shirts, they relayed stories of their own visit with the FDNY.

As a part of their own healing process, New York firefighters traveled to small firehouses located in the Blue Mountains. One group of them had a special request—their only one—to stand beside truck No. 343. That was the number of firefighters who lost their lives on 9-11.

Michael knocked, and a firefighter answered. Michael introduces himself. The firefighter shakes Michael's hand. He explains that it has become *too much* to trade shirts. Some firefighters do it individually, but as a group, they can no longer participate. He then politely directs Michael to another station ten blocks away who are more likely to be able to accommodate this request. It was a somber moment. Beneath the sorrow, I was glad to have witnessed that handshake between men who had committed themselves to the same goal, who cherished the same memory.

We played the *Charlie Brown Christmas Special* music on the CD player during our last evening in New York. This has been a city of many *firsts* for us. In this town, we chose our first pre-ordered turkey from the back of a truck in the Fairview Market where half of its produce was displayed on the sidewalk and the other half towered overhead down narrow aisles. It was our first holiday among frantic grocery shoppers, all vying for a prime spot to park their cart while they gathered the perfect apples for their pie, the perfect squash for their hot dish, the perfect cranberries for their relish—all in an effort to produce a meal to celebrate the Giving of Thanks.

In this market, Abigail notices for the first time that everyone around her appears pushy and impatient. I explained, "That's one of the marvelous things about this city. New Yorkers take pride in their ability to speak out to others around them. It represents their *rite of passage*." She nods. A passerby who has overheard my explanation smiles, as though to the truth behind my words to Abigail. My confirmation.

It is our seventh evening. We sat around the table, recounting our adventures and blessings. It is a perfect picture of gratitude. Michael and I were able to create a memory important to us but also important that we gave our children. As in *An Affair to Remember*, I had taken Michael to the top of the Empire State Building and told him that I chose him to live the rest of my life with. My children yelled, "Ahhhhh" and "Gross!" turning away in elaborate disgust from our kisses and hugs.

But they were smiling.

My contract with life has not been broken. This cancer adventure only enhanced it. It is true that the unexpected had come flying at us one March afternoon when my only thoughts were of planning Abigail's fifth birthday party. Now, thirty months later, we are still together, still whole in new ways.

I read, recently, that a young man has invented a new technique to clean and enhance the true colors of the Mona Lisa. Through this process, he had discovered that the original painting had been altered, changes that could affect centuries of interpretation of this famous painting.

"Her secret is about to be revealed," I think aloud. An artist paints because he or she needs to. Does the message to others mean all that much to the artist in the end? Perhaps not. Perhaps it is the process of discovery, whether it requires a single year or a century, that holds the meaning of the message.

Cancer permanently altered my life and the lives of those that shared it with me, but it didn't destroy my life or end it in any way. Rather, these past two years have given me gifts far exceeding anything that it took away.

What secrets did it reveal? I believe I am personally discovering these things. Like the Mona Lisa, however, the artist changed his mind periodically. The discoveries lay upon each other. Do we have a whole new painting to learn from? Or, perhaps, an old one with a new message?

My contract to live this life feels as if many addenda have been attached to it, but they have come with agreements to enhance and to enlighten it. It is a duty that I will gladly fulfill. I am grateful for my gifts of life. I watch Abigail's wonder as she notices that snowflakes change colors with music. I watch the gradual overwhelming of Benjamin, counting taxis in a city with an unending supply of the yellow cars.

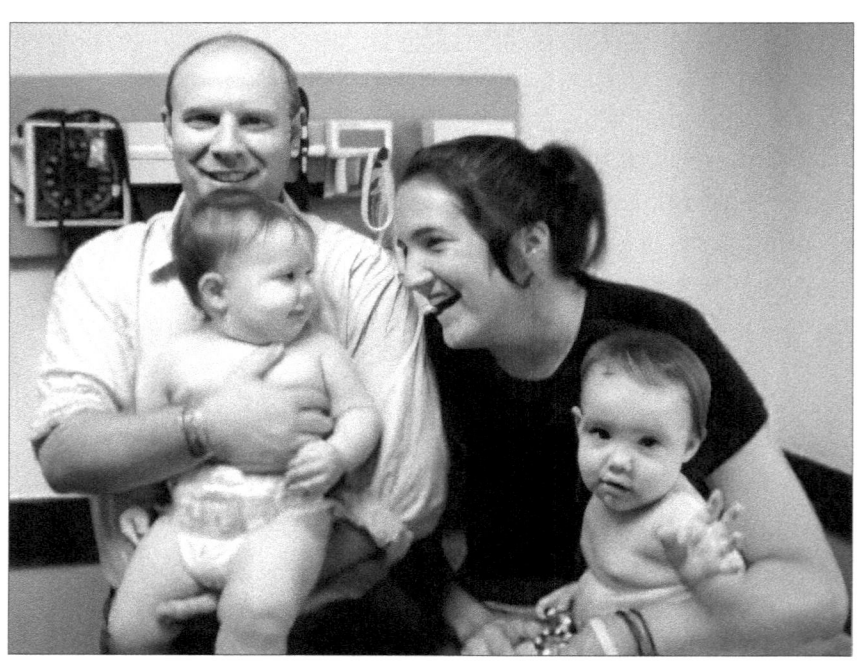

C is for "Community"

To love and be loved is to feel the sun from both sides.
—David Viscott

Communities of caring saved my family and me over and over and over during our cancer adventure. When I say *saved* I mean—picked up my kids from school when a chemo session ran late, fed us when we were too exhausted to cook at the end of a long day, flew across state lines to clean our home or take a walk with me. When my mind became the biggest obstacle to my inner peace, these acts of kindness eased my racing thoughts and let me simply manage the information that was *here and now* rather than traveling to the scary place of *what if. . ."*

Practicing yoga offered me a sanctuary where I could use my body to heal, rather than hurt. When the repeated penetration of needles violated my body, my mind and spirit reacted defensively, wanting to wrap around me to guard it against these intruders. To protect it.

Yoga brought me to this place of healing. I could be in a room full of people but hear only my own breathing. I could feel my sweat purging toxins, cleansing my body, wringing it out. In the end, after our final resting pose, life seemed better, not so dire.

I suddenly became aware of the community that surrounded me. I was always greeted with loving arms. No one there was ever shy or afraid of the physical changes they would see in me. Love is the remedy that heals. In this studio, I received the maximum dose I needed for the day.

One teacher in particular, Kim Dastrup, rarely saw my bald head or absent eyebrows. Not because they weren't conspicuous but because Kim didn't see what's missing, she only saw a person's heart and spirit. She greeted each of us with the sort of genuine enthusiasm associated with a dear friend we haven't seen for months. It is the kind of welcome that I longed for after a difficult day or before the beginning of a new one.:.

"Amy! How have you been? We need to talk. . ."

Kim greeted you in English or Italian. Either way it was a loving embrace. Very few people radiate this quality of affection and still maintain its integrity. She kept it genuine, authentic.

Her smile broadened, the glow intensifying when she greeted each student with her eyes. She radiated loving gratitude for this opportunity to practice together. She remembers everyone's name and often accompanies her greeting with a detail of their life or the next sentence in a conversation she started last week—and which will never end.

I believe she could run any company with her skills. She has mastered it. Yet she chooses yoga as her passion and aspires only to the honor the capacity of, *teacher*.

Kim interprets our body expression's while we practice. Whether that expression is pain, struggle, or joy, she was able to shape our practice so that it guided us through our transition from challenge to ease, from struggle to release.

In the end, we all celebrated as we approached our mats with happiness. The physical poses of yoga assist in revealing our deepest emotions, our inner being. Kim is an excellent translator.

I attended her class following my transfusions.

On Wednesday, I would have chemotherapy, and on Thursday I would have my Neulasta shot. This shot is pure science! Neulasta helps to restore all the white blood cells chemo has destroyed. But it made my body ache something awful. Even my hair would hurt—when I had some. It is also mighty expensive, seven thousand dollars an injection. I had seven of them.

Then, on Friday I would attend Kim's 8:30 AM yoga class. This was, typically, my *blue* day, but it would have been even more depressing if I didn't attend her class, so I made a promise to myself that no matter how I was feeling, I'd be there. The results far outweighed my physical and mental depression.

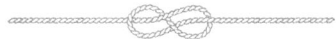

My four months of treatment were drawing to a close near the end of August 2005. Sarah came from out-of-state and attended Kim's class with me. She was the eighth, and last, person we had asked to come help us take care of the kids while Michael took care of me.

Friendships can be tried by inconvenient demands, but Sarah volunteered, even though she had twin two-year-olds and lived in a state where she had no immediate family around. Her mother-in-law flew from Michigan to Oklahoma to take care of the twins so that Sarah could fly from Oklahoma to Utah to take care of us. Sarah is a blessing in many respects, but this sort of commitment was the *hallmark* of her friendship.

I wanted to share Kim with her. At the end of class, Kim always came to each of us as we lie supine during Savasana, and she would rub our heads. Her touch is always welcoming. I look forward to this portion of the class each and every time. When the music has ended, and we bring our own hands to meet again to clasp in our heart space. We sit comfortably in cross-legged positions, and close our practice by bowing forward and saying,

"Namaste," a Sanskrit word that can be interpreted in many ways.

The meaning I like best is, *The light within me honors the light within you.*

I glanced over at Sarah, my eyebrows (the few hairs that were left) arched inquiringly about how she was doing.

 "I couldn't release my tension until Kim held my head, and then I found myself releasing everything. It was like magic."

I smiled. "I know exactly what you mean."

Coffee, Tea, and Community

No one is useless who has a friend,
and if we are loved we are indispensable.
—Robert Louis Stevenson

Some people may think of Salt Lake City only as the Mormon capital of the world with its own brand of community involvement. But there are communities within communities within communities of all faiths, non-faiths, yoga, school, skiing, hiking and, yes, coffee houses.

The Coffee Garden is located on the corner of 900 East and 900 South. *Ninth and Ninth* we call it. It was one of the first places friends took Michael and me when we were considering moving to Utah. It's a coffee shop co-owned by a kind man named Allen who spearheads this coffee community by simply offering a meeting place.

He once bought me a decaf mocha when I was about seventeen months pregnant with Benjamin; okay, nine months, but it felt like seventeen. I was feeling a desperate need to regain my body and birth this child. He handed over my drink, compliments of the house, with the hopeful wish, "Perhaps this will work."

Twelve hours later, my water broke and my Benjamin, all eight and half pounds of him, was born. Ten years later, I still thank Allen for that cup of coffee!

The Coffee Garden is a gathering place of artists, writers, businesspeople and yoga practitioners—a studio is just down the street. It is a community in itself. Recently, it relocated across the street from its original location but had to close its doors for four months of renovation.

The Coffee Garden community suddenly found itself without its bearings. Our internal GPS readings for a coffee community were bleeping helplessly. Coffee Garden people were sighted wandering the streets, looking for a place to hang out, corporate brand coffee cups in hand (a grievous failure as a substitute) to discuss their life's stories or play a game of chess. Laptop people searched for an outlet to plug in, only to tune out. And then, there were people like me, a newly converted tea drinker, all of us searching for our spot.

The Coffee Garden is a place where people, me included, find sanctuary. This is where I would meet with Kelly O'Reilly (my bandanna buddy who was going through treatment for lung cancer) and her husband, Joe, to discuss the purpose of our day. I often called Michael to join us. This collection of people who met in that familiar dwelling created a perfect environment for our husbands to chat, to share, and to compare notes of living through their own version of cancer. Of all of the places people could meet, this coffee spot was the one place we chose to assist us in facing our fears surrounding cancer.

For Michael and Joe, this place lived up to its name, Coffee Garden A nurturing place where we could grow.

Kelly and I often chatted without our husbands. We both felt concern for them, as they maintained course as we swerved in and out of it.

"Who is taking care of them?" we would ask each other. "We are," we would each confirm, aloud and silently. Kelly and I each shared this understanding of our husbands, our marriages, and our illness.

Kelly and I also held a strong connection to our own bodies. Practicing yoga only heightened our awareness of this connection. We each felt like a huge science experiment.

"A Petri dish!" I proclaimed myself to be. Biologically, we understood the demands that chemo was placing on our body. We each spoke about the ease of wrapping our brain around this concept.

What was—dare I say, fascinating? about our chemo-bodies was the way they responded to our yoga practice.

The wringing out of toxins from muscles.

A flushing or cleansing opened up the channels of energy

The exchange of *bad* for the *good*.

Kelly felt the effects especially in her lungs. Having never *felt* cancer, only the effects of the treatment, I experienced the yoga in my muscles and in the overall sense of well-being that followed. We each accepted yoga as a healing practice and strongly felt that it should be prescribed simultaneously with the toxic remedies.

These were our conversations, held in our welcoming coffee community meeting place. As we feasted on sweets or sipped our tea, it was the flow of conversation that supported our bond of friendship and offered a moment for us to support one another without self-pity or shame. We fed our souls simultaneously with our bellies. We warmed our hearts with tea and conversation.

When I found out I had cancer, I stopped drinking coffee and started drinking green tea. The Coffee Garden had a lovely variety of green teas for me to choose from, Jasmine Pearl, Sencha, and my favorite, Sky between the Branches. Even the sound of their names brightened my spirits. Once the baristas memorized my orders for coffee, they also memorized my orders for various teas. I loved their personalized service, remembering my name and my usual drink order.

One morning, well into my baldness, I stepped up to the counter to present the barista with my order. I was glowing from a good yoga practice and most surely was smiling. As was often the case, five-year-old Abigail was standing beside me when I placed my order, and the barista greeted us both with a smile.

"How are you doing?"

"I'm good today."

"Well," she said, "Today, your tea is on me."

I was taken back and touched at this kindness from a near-stranger.

"Thank you. That is very kind of you."

I looked down at Abigail, then back up to meet the barista's eyes. She, too, wore a bandanna. Her reasons were different from mine, but I was sure Abigail had noticed it.

It was this kindness of "strangers" that helped me to know that I was going to be okay.

Thank you.

Girlfriends Forever

A friend is someone who knows the song in your heart and can sing it back to you when you have forgotten the words.

—Unknown

It's not exactly a news flash, but girlfriends make the insanity of a situation appear sane. They make it possible to think clearly in chaos, to show up in a vacant room, to say the words that need to be said and hear those words with their whole being. To me, the bond that ties girlfriends to girlfriends is the secret glue known only to the estrogen-enhanced sex and, I believe, secretly sought after by men and the government.

You see, it's a bond that can solve world problems, soothe the Middle East, calm the Koreas, and ease the pain between China and Tibet. Girlfriends nurture this bond with rich servings of chocolate, wine, and espresso. Occasionally, it craves arugula, but it also chomps down on a good Swiss on rye.

Girlfriends see you through changes and accept most of them, except for those they can't stand, which they'll tell you about right away. It may end in a fight and a few deleted emails or abrupt text messages, but eventually you realize, "Ahhh, you were right." And you'll be grateful for their insight.

Girlfriends love all parts of you. They understand childbirth and hormonal changes. They know what it's like to be loved thoroughly and then want to be left alone for a time. They share the emotions that come with parenting, marriage, partners, or being single, and can empathize through a difficult divorce.

Girlfriends share strengths and doubts. They share their own doubts when their bodies fail them. They support and lift you when doubt presses down hard, replacing it with the presence of certainty.

After I finished a practice, I walked up the street to the Coffee Garden for a cup of tea. Whom do I see? My girlfriends! I hear them laughing even before I see them, gathered around a patio table golden streams of sunlight all around them.

One of our fellow survivors, TerriLyn, is describing a breast infection that required surgery. She is telling us about the experience when she and her mother were in the prep room.

The pre-surgical nurse instructed, "Take this marker and draw a circle around your breast with the infection."

"What?"

We all exchanged puzzled looks.

Karen asked, "Doesn't he know which one is infected? And why a marker?"

TerriLyn explains, "The surgeon doesn't want to make any errors."

Lyle said, "Yeah, I heard on the news about a patient who needed to have his leg amputated and the doctor removed the wrong leg."

We all gasped.

The nurse repeated mechanically to TerriLyn, "Take this marker and circle the breast that is of concern."

TerriLyn hesitantly took the pen. "Okaaay . . ."

She asked the nurse "Dr. Massey knows which one, right? I mean, the reason why I'm even here is because she wanted to make clean cuts so that it would finally heal."

The nurse didn't even blink. She shoved the marker into TerriLyn's hand. "Circle the breast that is of concern," she droned then left the room.

"Geez!" Disgusted, TerriLyn turned to her mother.

Trisha's eyes widened, "I can't believe it!"

A woman at the table next to ours looks over. I can tell she wants to join the conversation.

"Doesn't she know which one is infected? And why a marker?" Lyle asked again.

"That's dreadful!" said Deanne.

"A hospital is not an assembly line!" Lyle was fuming by now.

"I don't understand," says Marie, her voice calm. She is breast feeding her baby daughter. "How did we get to the point in the surgical world when a woman's infected breast has to be identified with a sharpie? Are doctors so out of touch with their patients that they need arrows pointing to the—what did she call it? The area of concern? Seriously, is medical care that distant from our bodies?

TerriLyn tells us that she found the perfect response. She took the marker from her mother. "Mom let's really make it obvious! *Really* obvious. Let's draw an eyeball around my breast."

"With eyelashes!" Terrilyn had continued.

Terrilyn's mom nodded enthusiastically. "And let's write a message! How about, 'I'm watching you!' or 'I'm keeping an eye on you!'"

They were both laughing when TerriLyn ripped open her hospital gown. Her mother took the marker and whipped off the cap.

The woman at the next table moved her chair a foot in our direction.

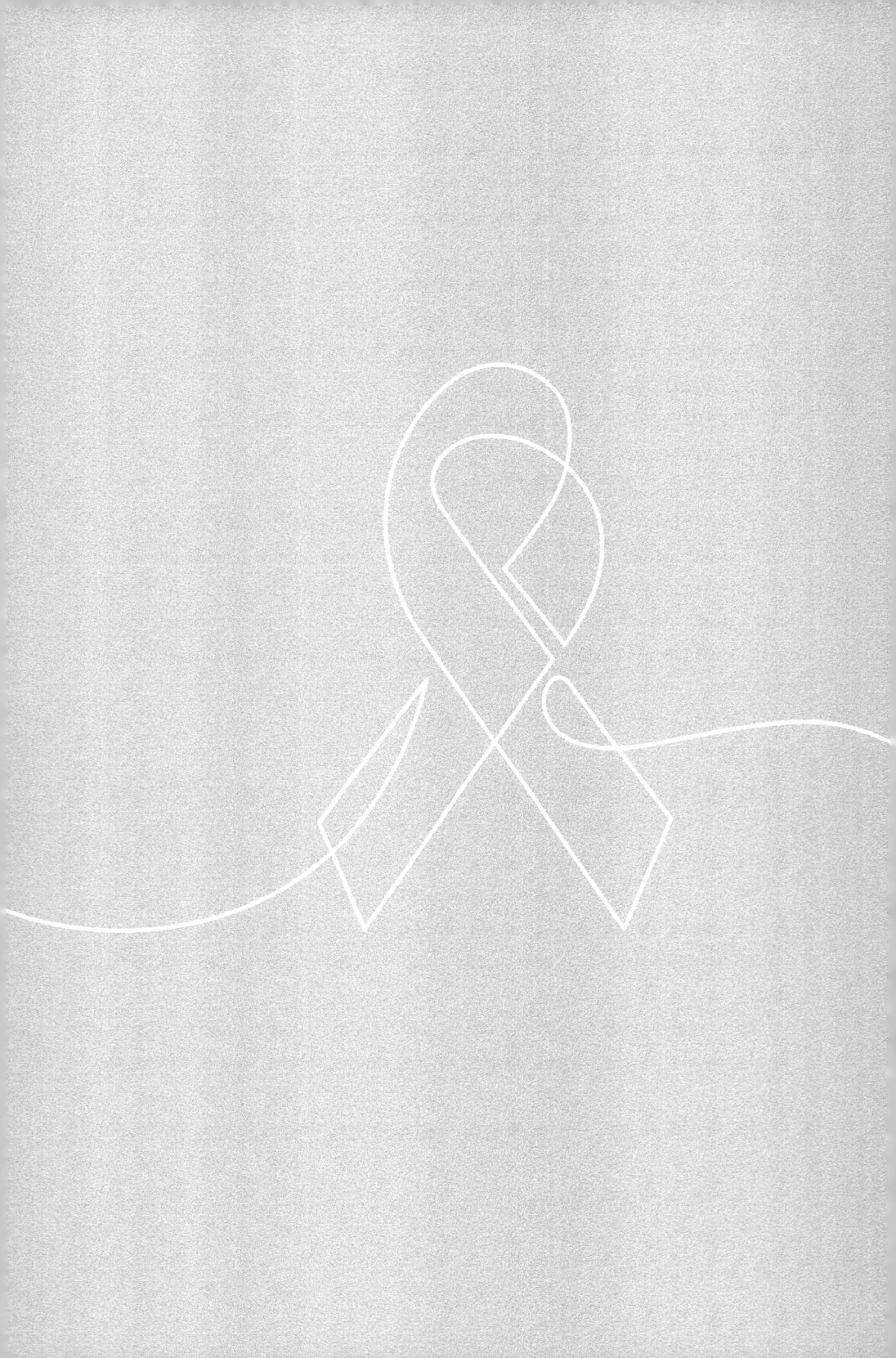

At the Oyster Bar with the Breast Cancer Girls

I haven't trusted polls since I read that 62% of women had affairs during their lunch hour. I've never met a woman in my life who would give up lunch for sex.

—Erma Bombeck

There are five of us, and we are gathered to celebrate Lauren's *most-nearly-well* day. Lauren is our friend from our school community. I met her in the classroom. Her daughter and my son shared a teacher.

In the fall of 2006, our teacher, knowing that I am a breast cancer survivor, asked if I would meet with Lauren; that she had some questions for me. Lauren held her one year old on her hip while we walked to the neighborhood coffee shop. She told me that while weaning her daughter from breastfeeding she discovered that only one breast recessed while the other breast remained engorged.

After a series of examinations, she was informed that she had a nine cm sized tumor in her breast. By Thanksgiving, she had a bi-lateral mastectomy and reconstruction and by Christmas she began her year-long series of chemotherapy treatments. Choosing good days were more troublesome than finding difficult ones.

We picked Lauren up at home, and went to the Oyster Bar, her favorite restaurant. Then we showered her with gifts for *no reason* except for the mere fact that she was surviving. And wasn't this a good enough reason for celebrating?

Her husband and children, a third grader and now, an eighteen-month-old, met us at the door. Lauren was getting ready. Bubbly and ecstatic, she came from around the fireplace that was located in the center of the living room. The sun was setting, and golden beams streamed through the windows.

She walked into that golden glow. Everyone was smiling. It was such a pleasure to do this for her. Her husband told us, "She never goes out with the girls." Then he thanked us for celebrating her *one day of wellness*.

Lauren received weekly treatments for her HER2+ diagnosis. (HER2 stands for Human Epidermal growth factor Receptor 2. HER2+ tumors tend to grow and spread more quickly than tumors that are not HER2+. In addition, the treatment of HER2+ breast cancer is different than the treatment of breast cancer that is not.)

The timeline from diagnosis to surgery to treatment will take eleven months, which does not include reconstructive surgery and post-treatment medications. Eleven months of hospital transfusions. Due to her weekly Thursday transfusions, Wednesday is the only day she felt herself. So, we took her out to the Oyster Bar on Wednesday, her choice.

Three of us drove with Lauren. The fifth friend met us there. Electricity that was in the air, in the car, on the sidewalk, in the restaurant, and around our table was so contagious I just knew that other people in the room wanted to belly up and join in.

Our laughter was continuous!

Lauren had told us appetizers were fifty percent off before 6:00 p.m., so we ordered every appetizer on the menu and a couple of bottles of wine. Our conversation wove the fabric of our daily lives without one mention of a hospital or a treatment protocol. The five of us had a total of eleven children, the oldest eight years of age. We accepted that there were no guarantees in what we had been blessed with. But to waste any of that time was simply not the way to live.

With the wine remaining in our glasses, we uttered our defiant toast, "To life!"

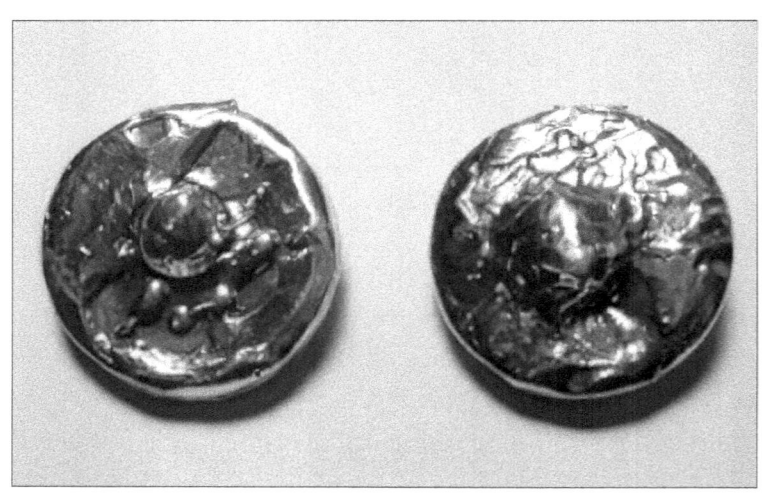

Casting Party

Although the world is full of suffering,
it is full also of the overcoming of it.

—Helen Keller

A gathering of women, some survivors, some caregivers, some just friends who care. We came together to support our friend, Laura, an artist. We agreed to help her make jewelry for her show *Thickening the Skin: A Tribute to Women with Breast Cancer.*

My friend, Kim, telephoned before coming over, warning me that she couldn't stay long but wanted to make a showing to support all of us. She arrived first—exactly on time, announced that she had a headache, and asked if she could contribute to the cause and then leave.

She ended up staying two hours and enjoyed every minute of it. Her headache? I'm not sure where it went.

The energy of friendship took over, it consumed us all.

Gratitude.

I was always amazed that women could take off their shirts to reveal their authentic self. We were an eclectic group. One young woman had difficulty sharing the fact that she lost her mom to breast cancer. Some women had eating disorders who struggled with body image. Some were extroverts, who had no difficulty disrobing in front of others.

Some did. But all of us embraced that moment in time. This cause. This rite of passage. We released the thing that we feared the most. Secrets shown. Not displayed but shared. A sacred space of womanhood and friendship.

One woman had no nipples, just *a mound*, the doctors called it. Her reconstruction wasn't yet completed. The secret was breasts not quite fully reconstructed. Her mastectomy scar was her gift. Her's to share.

Our body types were as unique as the women themselves. After all, no two breasts were alike. Often one breast didn't even match the other only three inches away.

Laura casted our breasts, wax moldings of our nipples which were carved and used as a mold for sterling silver. When finished, the casted nipples were the size of a silver dollar, made to be worn on a chain around the neck. Laura decided to take the impression of the incomplete reconstructed breasts (with the missing nipples) and made them broader—not petite, and round in shape after all. Her breast impression was not circular. Rather, they were a road map of a process in action.

The reality was that Laura's art presented only the beauty of her work. It was not off-putting at all. The imprint of our skin was on the inside of the piece. A reflection of ourselves. A transcript. Our trademark. The outside is a beautiful piece of silver carved in a circle, weighted nicely to hang perfectly around the neck.

Laura wore such a piece from a woman who saved her nipple in the form of this art piece when she had a double mastectomy at age twenty-three. Sustained and cherished in a form carried around her neck rather than worn on her chest. Alive today, Laura's friend has expressed overwhelming joyfulness in surviving her cancer yet, she lives with implants and has expressed sadness that she will never be able to breast-feed her future babies. The pendant Laura wears reminds' all of us that breast cancer knows no boundaries and does not discriminate by age.

Each of us took a turn, shared food lovingly made from scratch, drank wine, and listened to Joni Mitchell.

"Chick music," Michael complained.

"Damn right!"

We laughed a lot. One by one, we disrobed and lay on Laura's yoga mat. She had us rub ice cubes on our breasts. We screamed and giggled from the shock of the cold.

"Amy, you didn't tell me about the ice," someone accused.

I shrugged. "It's art." I hadn't known about it either.

When Laura had explained her project to my A Quality Life Community class and asked for volunteers, I didn't hesitate. "I'm in."

The ice made our nipples harden. Followed by three ladles of non-toxic heated wax for each breast. Out of all of the experiences my nipples had been through, this was a first for them. My breasts had long belonged to others; my husband, my nursing babies, my doctors, and now an artist who immortalized them in sterling silver.

I felt as if my breasts had contributed to the breast cancer cause, rather than be removed for it. Full circle. The cycle of life. They gave, then I had parts of them removed, then they gave again. No other part of my body has contributed in this way to society.

"Be sure to capture my dimple," I told Laura. It marked the site of my lumpectomy. I felt good. A part of me had been molded and carved into sterling silver. This had never happened to me before. Ah, perhaps it did not happen *to me* but rather *for me*.

Yes. Yes.

Laura and the owner of the gallery had each agreed to a twenty percent donation of sales to our A Quality Life Community yoga class for cancer survivors, caregivers, and loved ones. Their contribution would be the first financial donation the class had received since I started it in 2006. Laura mentioned to me that her life was saved once, spared, and given a second chance. She considered this offer a gesture of *paying it forward*. This was her opportunity. She practiced yoga to remind her of her healthy lifestyle and not of the one that almost destroyed her.

Her desire to live inspired our desire to thrive.

Walking Angels

*Neither a lofty degree of intelligence nor imagination
nor both together go to the making of genius.
Love, love, love, that is the soul of genius.*

—Wolfgang Amadeus Mozart

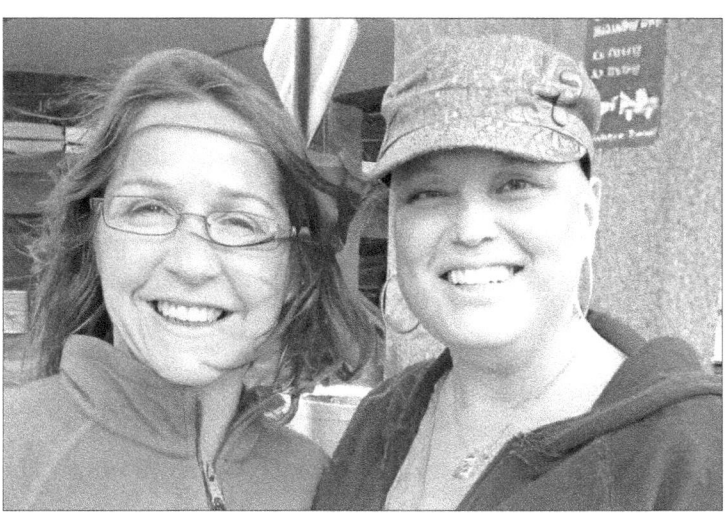

TerriLyn and I often talked about our encounters with *walking angels*. She told me about meeting one in a mall with her nine-year-old daughter, Isabella.

TerriLyn was feeling particularly low that day, chemo was taking a vicious toll on her emotions and afflicting her with periodic chemo-induced hot flashes. She was wearing a bandanna over her bald head. Both of them were waiting for something tangible to leap out and yell, "Buy me!"

"Perhaps a new pair of earrings?" she half-asked her daughter. It was the second part of her real question,: "What would make me feel better right now?"

A woman approached TerriLyn and her daughter, face glowing and eyes bright. She seemed familiar, but TerriLyn couldn't place her.

Without thinking she asked, "Do I know you?"

"No." The woman shook her head. "But I just wanted to say that you are looking great!"

TerriLyn was stunned "Thanks. Thank you very much." she stammered.

Then the woman was gone.

TerriLyn stood in the aisle looking down at Isabella. She ran her hand through her daughter's hair, then rested a hand on Isabella's shoulder. She appeared to be growing taller by the minute.

She looked more deeply into her daughter's face. Not surprised, not asking questions, just looking at her. She glanced again at the display, feeling a bit lighter than she had before this encounter. She smiled, "Isabella, wanna buy some earrings?"

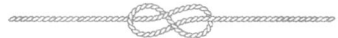

My family and I were in Las Vegas over Easter vacation visiting my husband's ninety-one-year-old Aunt Petris or *Auntie*. Who, by the way, acted nothing like a *typical* nonagenarian.

She gambled until 4:00 a.m., drank beer when she wanted to, and faithfully went to church on Sundays. Okay, maybe church is *typical*.

We liked to visit her over Easter because this is when she *graduates* from Lent. For six weeks, she gives up her vices, gambling, chocolate, and beer. On Easter morning, she rises for the sunrise service—probably the only dawn she has seen since last Easter's. She is not a morning person.

After visiting with Auntie, our kids clamor to see the Stratosphere or what we fondly call, *The Tower of God*. Traveling up a thousand feet, three floors per second, as the elevator operators dutifully report, we reach the observation floor and gaped at the view.

Vegas is considered *Sin City*. But from a thousand feet up, there are many beautiful sites revealing their panoramic secrets. Red rocks rise up on the outskirts of the bowl encasing the city, providing a deep nourishing backdrop.

I rode my bike, hiked to waterfalls with my children, and rock-climbed the red cliffs with my husband. It's odd. You don't often associate natural beauty with a town that places its emphasis on facades. But the rocks are real, and surely some of the people who travel to *sin city* are real too.

The rides on top of the *Tower of God* are scary as hell. Big Shot, Insanity Ride, and the X-Stream. Everyone in line is trying to talk everyone around them out of participating, yet they all go, and then they all buy the photos. In the end, they all love that they went.

But one woman was different. We met her on the speedy three-floor-per-second elevator ride. Don't get me wrong. She anticipated fear and showed it. She was, after all, human. However, both Michael and I clearly sensed something more in her.

She was willing to face this challenge, and it was her courage we noticed. Everybody else in line was broadcasting their fears while smiling nervously and digging their fingernails into their spouses' biceps.

This lady was with a woman friend, holding onto her arm. The friend was radiating fear, panic, and terror with the rest of us. But our woman was smiling—a beautiful, glowing smile, foregrounded against the distant background of these rich red rocks. She clearly knew the direction she was headed.

Her hair was styled short with tiny spikes on top; it seemed to fit her sassy personality. The weather was warm even for spring in Las Vegas, and she was wearing a tube top.

Visible, above the edge of this top was the telltale circular bump of a recently implanted *port-a-cath*, a catheter implanted below her left collarbone so that medication could be administered directly into her heart and pumped quickly throughout her body. It told us she was about to start chemotherapy.

Michael and I looked at each other. Suddenly and simultaneously, we understood everything. She had cut her the hair short before it fell out, exposing the surgical incision so that it would heal faster, but most of all, facing her fear full front by doing something that scared the socks off everybody else—and all of it with the most beautiful smile on her face. Her friend was leaning on her for support.

We saw their photographs after they had completed the X-Scream ride, a car teetering on railed tracks over the edge of the Stratosphere tower. The passengers ride in pairs, with four rows per car. The platform extends approximately thirty feet, half of it extending beyond the tower, a thousand feet off the ground. This ride was so terrifying that we didn't ride we only took pictures. Sure enough, of the passengers in her car, she was the only one who had her eyes open to anticipate the adventure and who wore a confident expression in anticipation of the results.

There, a thousand feet off the ground, I knew I was meeting a walking angel. She seemed to know she was in for the ride of a lifetime and that it was going to consume some of her energy reserves for a while, most likely drawing other angels, to *reboot* her. Yet her confidence was recognizable and contagious. I was proud of her bravery and was honored to have been in her presence for the brief moments of our ascent over a glittering city with the glorious red rocks as our backdrop.

Does this happen to other people besides TerriLyn and me? I've told one story about each of us, but the experience isn't unique. I wish we'd kept a better log of those moments when strangers approached us, briefly engaged us in uplifting and motivating conversation, and then they would disappear, never to be seen again, but leaving behind their positive energy and the realization that we desperately needed that exchange to get through the day.

Did we call it to happen? Was it a higher source that was taking care of us all along? Regardless of our belief systems, there were too many to be coincidental—happening at just the right place at just the right moment—when we needed them.

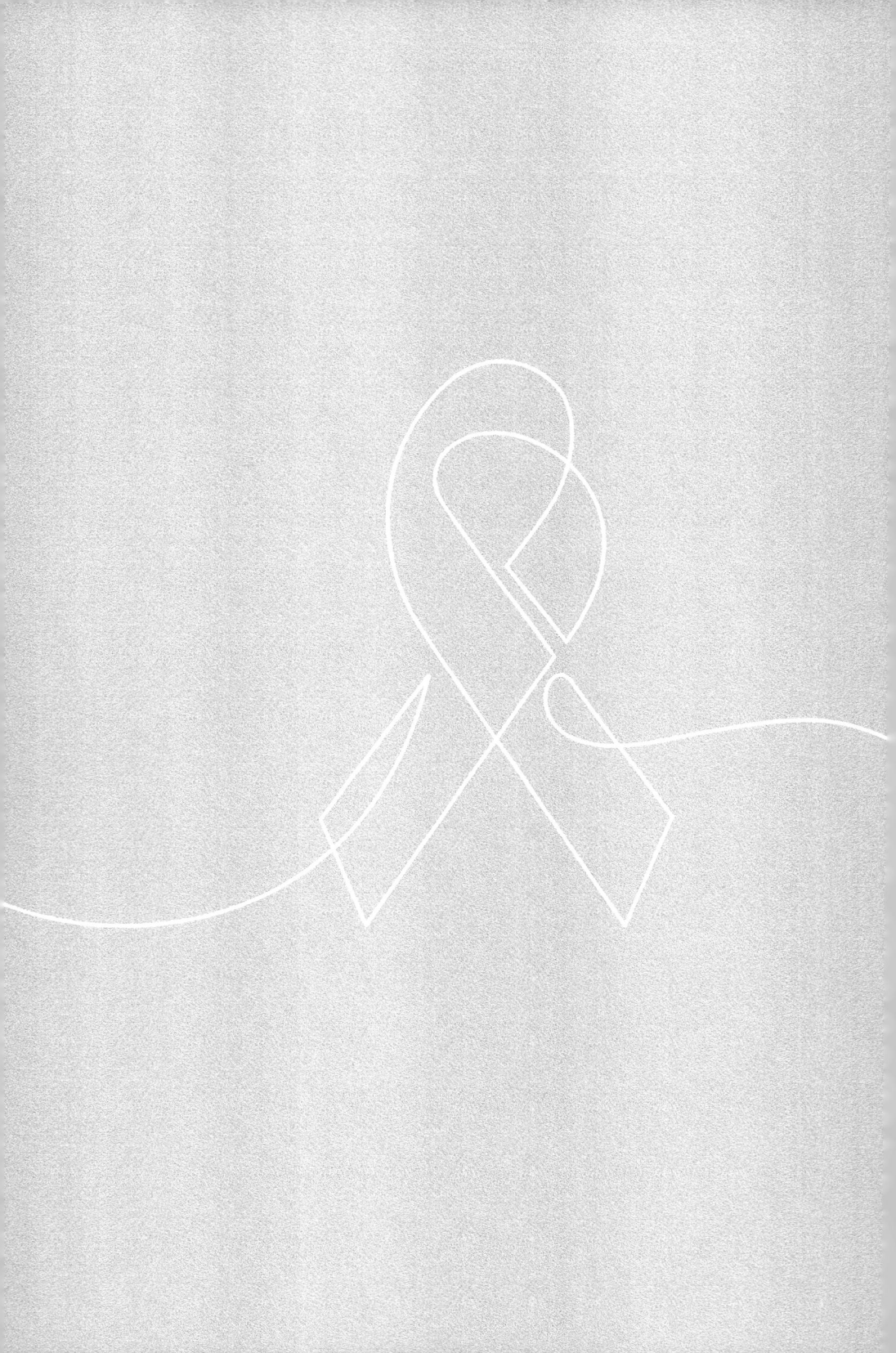

The Numbers Game

When we face the worst that can happen in any situation, we grow. When circumstances are at their worst, we can find our best.
—Elizabeth Kubler-Ross

Every month now, I meet a new person with cancer. These women and men are all under age forty. It feels like an epidemic.

A mother under forty walked up the stairs to the yoga studio last Saturday. She walked up the same steps this Saturday. Only this time she was bald.

"What's going on?"

She holds her eighteen-month-old on her hip; her four-year-old daughter is here to take my Yoga Kids class. She was dressed for yoga too.

"Breast cancer."

I ran into the office and returned, book in hand. I gave it to her. *Meditations from the Mat* by Rolf Gates. I tell her about our A Quality Life Community workshops and weekly Thursday night classes.

The yoga class I run at A Quality Life Community for cancer survivors, caregivers, and their loved ones, is free because our motto is, *Bringing Wellness to Life.*

In this class I meet people who share a common experience that I am able to connect to. We share common ailments, treatments, doctors, wellness, and fears. Many of us have young children, so we share a common and fierce drive to survive.

"It's the kids," she tells me. "I don't know if I can attend on a school night because of the kids."

I told her that I understood. I wrote important dates in the book for her, of classes she should attend, if possible.

She looks scared. I've already noticed that her daughter wears her thoughts on her face. So does this woman. I know she is battling the fear of breast cancer.

"Where are you in your treatments?"

Young *yoginis* attending the kid's class and their parents eagerly sign in and encircle us. It seems odd to be holding this conversation in the midst of such chaos, but is the news of cancer ever non-chaotic? She mistakes the question for a request to report on her stage and grade—something I never asked my fellow survivors.

I quickly clarify my request. In my mind, the stage doesn't matter. It is the wellness that I seek.

She answers the clarified question, "I've just finished my second round."

"Okay. I'm here every Thursday night. And if I'm not here, there's a skilled sub. The workshops are opportunities to seek a deeper understanding of wellness within our bodies through the medium of yoga."

I encouraged her to attend by simply providing her with the dates.

It's time to go. I need to teach her daughter laughter. Mom needs to learn to move with her breath. We retreat to our separate classes but return an hour later, each feeling much better. I bid them both good-bye. They descend the stairs. I watch them open the door and light falls into the stairwell. The door swings shut, and its dark again.

I expect to see her the following week. But the very next morning, she emails me. She will be attending the Thursday night classes and the next workshop.

I write back, "You are brave and strong."

Is it the *mother bear* spirit deep within us that seeks to find the answers to our diagnosis? Is it fear? Whatever the motivation, my class is filled with women under forty with bald heads. They are fierce survivors who roar in warrior poses and surrender in the savasana pose. They seek release—but on their terms.

I used to think of forty as an age that was in the middle—between what seemed old and what seemed young. Middle-aged. Women who become pregnant at this age usually refer to these pregnancies as *oopsies*, but that paradigm is shifting.

My Catholic neighbor had two of these. I saw her, a newborn in her arms, at the high school graduation ceremony of her oldest son. Eighteen months later, she gave birth again. Maybe it was intentional, to give the first child a friend. That was exactly what happened. They took care of each other. The four older children, all strategically spaced two years apart, all graduated rhythmically from high school, then college. By the time, the first *oopsie* entered first grade, the oldest brother was bringing home his own newborn to greet, share, and carry on with family traditions. This was my strongest association about women who turn forty, things don't go quite as they were planned.

Soon after, the number forty started meaning the sandwich generation. Not eating sandwiches, just feeling like one. Being sandwiched between two *needy* generations—parents who are no longer independent and may require nursing assistance or help to continue living independently. And then the children, learning independence but falling short of it.

Caring for the two slices of the sandwich often falls upon

women, who are often near forty. Where is such a woman's identity? Does it simply transfer to those for whom she is caring? Has she lost her dreams and desires? Was she ever given the opportunity to even formulate them? Perhaps not, her life appears fairly busy. Busy taking care of others or nurturing other lives. *Busy* can take years until her number is no longer forty.

I now know the number forty as the age when my peers and I are just completing the breast feeding of the final child. We have completed our college degrees. We have traveled—sought out sites in Europe, lived on a commune in Virginia, followed the Grateful Dead cross-country, and juggled for a panhandler's living in the Haight.

After, what I call, this *post-graduate-pre-adulthood* period of our lives, my peers and I have, individually, found our loves, our soul mates, the men with whom we dance to Frank Sinatra music. One fantastic wedding ceremony later, everyone from graduate school with the mates included, careers begin for some, babies are born for others, perimenopause begins for some of us. And here the cycle ends where this paragraph began, breast feeding.

Or does it?

The one thing that was never on the forty-year plan was the lump. My OB-GYN, five months pregnant at forty, herself, while assisting me in delivering my second child, tells me that, once the baby hormones leave my body, there will be a good chance that early stages of menopause will begin. I just looked at her.

Well, at least we'll be going through this together.

But the lump thing. Um, this was not in the plan. Sore knees, early stages of arthritis from too many marathons on asphalt, lower back pain, too many long bike rides up and down canyon roads through our beautiful mountains, crow's feet on the outskirts of my eyes. Yes, these are things I expected to start showing up along with the number forty.

But not the lump.

"I have a thirteen-month-old!" My student blasts.
"I have a four-year-old daughter!" Says another.
"I have a life to live and children to raise!"
We all expound with mighty fists raised to the sky.

We, collaboratively, are clearly not done. My class is filled with women who simply come with questions, "Why? Why the lump? And how? There is no history of breast cancer in my family. What is going on?"

Could it be the complexity of this woman and her number? She is an educated woman, is a mother, and holds down a career. She is a manager of household activities. She is a partner to her soul mate.

"She's bringing home the bacon and frying it up in the pan!"

She's the woman that Helen Reddy sang about. She's also one weary woman, hitting the pillow as soon as the children do.

Has this superwoman evolved into yet another version of the motherhood role? Or has she only tacked more onto the duties created by her predecessors? Have the forty-year-olds created such an environment that there is no room to breathe? No place to vent? No time to exhale, to release?

Could it be that, perhaps, through some sort of personalized crazy internal warning device that this is where the lump is created?

That's nuts! I exhale! I practice yoga four times a week! I schedule it after dropping one kid off at school and before picking up the other one from music class while simmering a delicious veggie stew in my crock pot for dinner which will finish cooking while I tutor three students after school. Internalizing? Hmpf, right! You know, it's got to be something in the water or in the air! After all, we do have holes in the ozone!

Regardless of the cause, it's still a lump and it wasn't in the master plan, damn it.

So, here is the next plan, Cure it! When I began running

in the *Salt Lake City Race for the Cure,* it started at the Capitol. Three hundred people showed up and we ran through the mountains. It was a glorious morning run, we all finished with honor, and we were each awarded a medal on a ribbon to be carried around our necks and over our hearts. Eleven years later, these same forty-year-olds are pushing their babies in running strollers and with lumps in their breasts. And now there are sixteen thousands of them.

I have found it fascinating that it is the *sick* who fight the hardest.

Today, I am joined by my peers, still with our soul mates beside us, with our children in tow, with our careers and our exercise classes, and still with our stiff knees and our lower back pain. But I'm also joined with them in a community of survivability. This law of attraction draws us together daily. It is this race that we all are given the opportunity to win. The number forty. It is a number that I am immensely proud of!

Four women under the age of forty at my school have been diagnosed with breast cancer. The stats are down from one in eight to one in seven. But why are women being diagnosed younger and younger? In radiation we talk about it. It's not an old ladies' disease anymore. Is it better screening? But women aren't encouraged to get a mammogram before age forty.

Is it education? Self-exams? Our environment? The food we eat. Yet my whole family said that I was the healthiest that they have ever known me to be.

Cancer has no boundaries. It travels across all playing fields in the game we call life. Michael says I'm too metaphorical.

Well, folks, here's the thing. The only number I have ever cared about—for my own diagnosis and with all of those whom I have met—is the number ninety.

That's the number of candles I'd like to see on my birthday cake.

Being "Pro-Active"

In rivers, the water that you touch is the last of what has passed and the first of that which comes, so with present time.
—Leonardo Da Vinci

"How do you know whether to believe or challenge your doctor? Is it possible to do both?"

A student in my yoga class had undergone treatment for ovarian cancer. Her test for BRCA 1 & 2 indicated positive. (BRCA are inherited alterations in the genes called BRCA1 and BRCA2, short for breast cancer 1 and breast cancer 2. They are involved in many cases of hereditary breast and ovarian cancer).

She had a young daughter and feared for her future. She wanted to heal her body on all levels, but what could she do with the fear? Her doctors told her to take anti-depressants. She did. It helped, but it did not offer what she was looking for to manage her fear. She wanted to feel her way toward healing, not just managing her illness.

She asked with sincerity, "How can I be *pro-active* in this situation? Which direction should I take?"

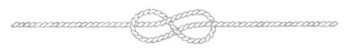

One evening my friend, Emma Jackson, called about 10:30 PM. She wanted to donate to A Quality Life Community and had a couple of questions. But in the end, she just needed to talk. She was a breast cancer survivor, too, and was one of the women I had originally called when I sought advice about treatment, alternative remedies, and raising children in the middle of it all. She helped me through a difficult time, and I will always be grateful to her. However, I suddenly became aware that the tables had shifted, and I was no longer the inquirer.

Emma was seeking advice, and I had become her ear.

She told me that she found herself becoming increasingly depressed. She had landed in a hole and wanted to climb out of it. She inquired about a support group—people who understood and perhaps shared her frustrations. She missed her active body and suddenly found herself concerned with being a single-breasted woman. It had been more than three years since her diagnosis, but those thoughts and feelings were just now surfacing.

I asked her, "What triggered this?"

She explained that she was due for a mammogram and had asked a physician friend about getting a more thorough evaluation, essentially an MRI. She understood that MRIs can give "false positives" and are costly, but she still decided to do it. Her friend made the appointment at a reputable hospital. She filled out the paperwork in triplicate, endured the time-consuming MRI procedure, and the frustration as nurses tried repeatedly to find hydrated veins to start her IV. We finished each other's sentences about the feeling that the pain is less important than the feeling that our bodies are failing us.

Two months later, she went in for her quarterly check-up and asked her oncologist, "So, what were the results of my MRI?"

Looking confused, her doctor shuffled through the file. No MRI results. She assured Emma that she would locate them. "They must not yet had arrived to be filed," her doctor construed.

Being "Pro-Active"

Emma left the office not knowing her test results.

Four months later, she was due for another mammogram. Emma's radiologist asked, "So, why didn't you have the MRI?"

Stunned, my friend responded with angst and urgency all at the same time. A wave of emotion flooded her as the last six months raced through her mind.

Questions like, "Was I not acting proactively? Was I not monitoring myself properly?" The first rule of cancer survivorship is self-advocacy, being proactive, pushing the envelope with most of our doctors.

Don't be afraid to ask questions.

After much investigation and insistence, Emma's MRI results were found on a shelf in the hospital, detached from any patient information. Apparently, the paperwork filled out in triplicate went in a different direction. Forwarded to her oncologist, the results indicated an area "of concern" in her remaining breast.

That was where my friend began to spiral down, feeling that she had dropped the ball, let down her defenses and let this happen to her. Thinking that she failed to follow through with her doctors more assertively.

All of the *coulda—shoulda—woulda's* ran through her mind. What aggravated her the most, however, was not her own lack of *proactivity* care but the chilling fact that a twenty-two thousand dollars test indicated a problem with the remaining breast of a breast cancer survivor and that it had been sitting on a shelf in a reputable and well-managed hospital for six months (*6 months!*) Why didn't anyone try to find who this test belonged to?

My friend had paid her bill, so the test results were not withheld due to an unpaid bill. This was an act of negligence. A reputable physician who was also her friend had recommended this hospital because it had the newest machines, the latest technology, the best-trained technicians.

She wavered between anger and heavy-heartedness.

"Amy, I understand that a hospital is a busy place, but these employees chose to work in these jobs. They should have shown more concern."

My friend is a kind-hearted, generous soul without a self-centered bone in her body. For this judgment to have been passed through her mind, let alone her lips, was an indication of how upset she was.

Suddenly, the past three years disappeared, and her year of treatment was the only thing she saw. The year of surgery, chemo, and radiation. She was overwhelmed with dread and a sense of failure. The fear was back, the confidence gone. Cancer had moved back into her house. How could she go through all of that again?

This was becoming all too familiar.

The mammogram. It was not sensitive enough for some diagnoses, but it was for others. Researchers work to refine its technical and mechanical sensitivity. Yet, the mammogram procedure, in its' existing state of technical sensitivity determines the next step of treatment—dismissal or more tests? This protocol alienates some people because they fear positive results, yet it also eliminates fear for others by providing clear negative results.

With Emma's remaining breast pressed between two plastic plates in various directions for optimum viewing, she endured temporary discomfort. We try to console ourselves, *it'll be over in a few minutes*, but the thought welled up, *it's just the beginning of discomfort*.

The downward spiral continued.

The tech announced, "The test results have been read. The doctor will see you in a moment to explain to you the results."

Like an old TV re-run that didn't get good ratings to begin with, my friend sat in her hospital gown in the tiny waiting room, thumbing outdated and hopelessly cheerful women's magazines. She faced a mirror directly in front of her. The gown bulged, or lay flat, in familiar places across her chest. Her face reviewed what was in her heart.

The familiar knock on the door.

She regained her composure, and lifted her chin, "Come in."

Emma was raised in the south. Dignity at all times, at all costs. She faced her radiologist, ready for the news, whatever it may be. She had two pre-teen sons and a husband who loved her. There was much to live for, much to fight for.

The radiologist was smiling. "You're clear to go."

And just like that, her life had once again taken an unexpected turn. After much explanation, apology, a promise to follow-up and follow through, Emma found herself in her car where tears welled up in her eyes.

What was the lesson behind this experience?

"I need a support group," she told me. "It's been three years and I think I'm finally ready."

If anyone could relate to a breast cancer survivor patient-advocate better, it would be a bunch of chest-compromised ex-patient survivors.

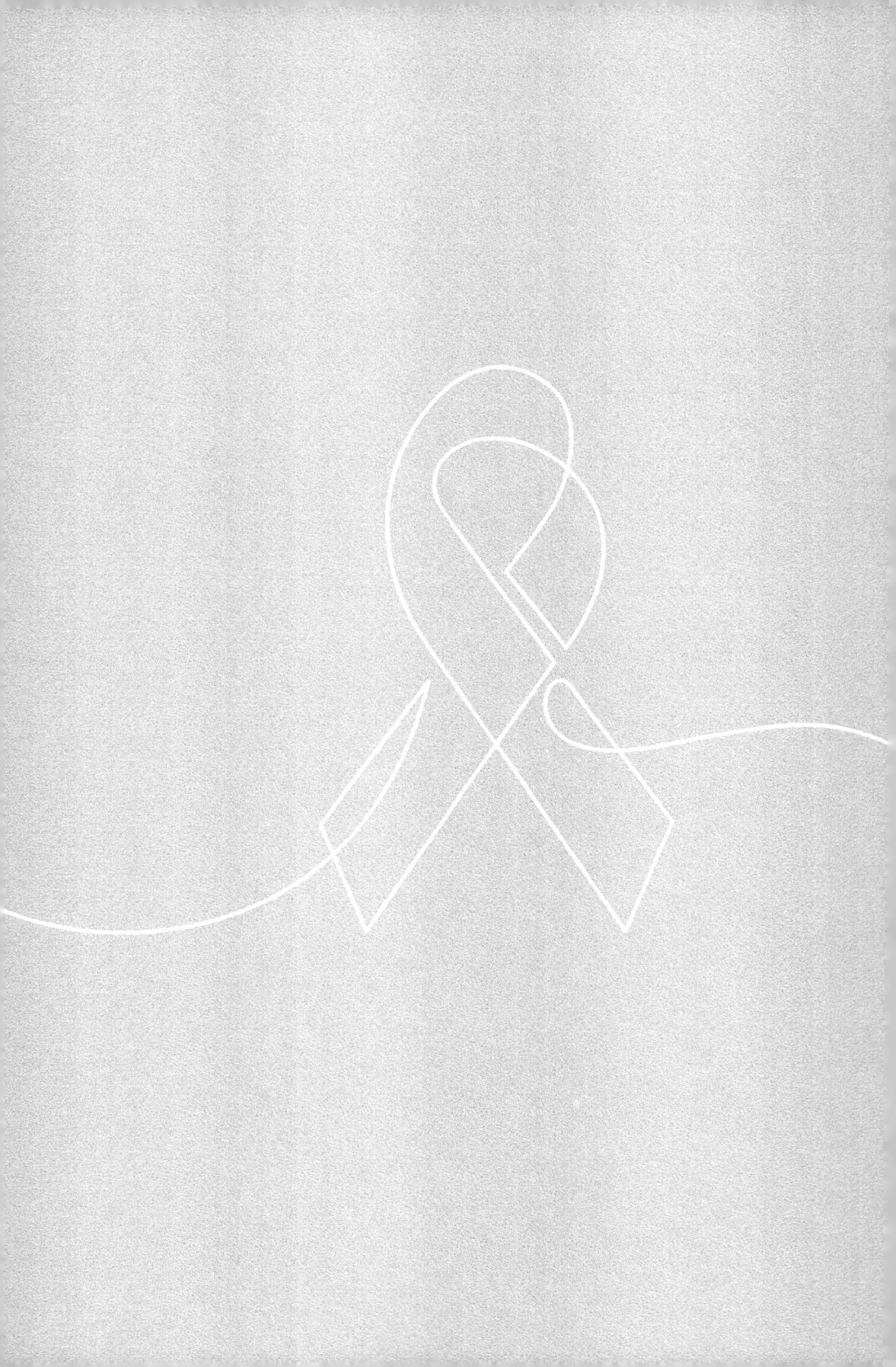

Being Capable

*We all have the extraordinary coded within us,
waiting to be released.*

—Jean Houston

Neurologists and infectious disease specialists can wrap their brains around breast cancer cerebrally, medically, and physically, but often forget to balance the emotional and spiritual side of cancer.

Healing has to be a well-rounded activity.

Capable women believe they can handle difficult circumstances. I know I believe this about myself. "I'm capable."

Yoga has taught me to challenge my inner independence. Yoga, during the time I was having cancer treatments, showed me that being vulnerable wasn't the same as being incapable. This was an important lesson for me. Placing my body in challenging poses, releasing muscles, opening my heart space, unlocking energy blocks—it all sounds so *hocus pocus* except for one thing—*it works*.

Witnessing my brave friends confirmed this conviction once again. It's not that we women undergoing cancer treatment aren't up for the challenge, or strong enough, or brave enough. It's just that we're now becoming aware that it's not overpowering this disease that heals us.

It's bringing it into a balance. Body, mind, and spirit. Balance.

Noticing Sunsets Again

The world connects not by molecules. It connects through ideas, hopes, faces, dreams, actions, stories, and memories.

—Barrie Stanford Greiff

In early June 2006, our family decided on a trip to Australia. It had been a little over a year since my diagnosis. The trip was our reward for surviving our cancer adventure together. But *saying* we were going to Australia and then actually making it happen are two different things.

Airline tickets alone would cost about four (4,000) thousand dollars—pretty steep for salaries of a teacher and a firefighter.

So, we asked for magic, and magic is what we got.

I was tutoring students after school from all over downtown Salt Lake City. I had worked with Sumner for over six years. When I submitted my invoices to his grandmother, I included a letter updating her on his progress, and I usually added tidbits about my family and me.

As matter of courtesy with all of my clients, I kept them informed about my situation His grandmother and I became close. She expressed concern in her return letters.

One day, she sent a check that paid for Sumner's entire year of tutoring services plus some extra *just because* cash. That check covered our airfare plus a little left over for travel expenses.

Magic.

While we were in Australia, my friend Erin, substituted my classes at A Quality Life Community yoga class. We visited friends in Sydney and Melbourne whom we had not seen since our honeymoon eleven years earlier, I kept in contact with Erin by email.

One evening I logged on and received a lengthy email. It was a suspenseful, step-by-step account of what had occurred the night before in the class.

> It was a warm evening and the swamp cooler had not yet been prepped. The room could only be cooled down by opening a window. The class was a good size, approximately ten people, which contributed to the rising temperature.

Barb, a fifty-something woman, was attending her second session. I was already smiling. Barb and her friend Gloria are a two-person mutual support unit. They proclaim themselves to be the "peanut gallery," a self-deprecatory phrase that positions them as observers. It's a ruse. They are participants, full participants. Each is funny as an individual, but together, they are hysterical.

I keep reading.

> I'm standing at the front of the mat with eyes closed and hands at the heart center, feet at hip bones distance apart, breathing in and out through the nostrils of the nose . . .

Erin's slowly divulging details was killing me!

What, Erin!? What happened?

I'm reading this in my friend's study. Their home is in a beautiful neighborhood just outside downtown Melbourne. I practically stopped breathing. I could visualize the scene all too clearly; the heat of the room, and the street noises through the open window. I know all ten of the people who were in attendance that evening.

> I heard a terrible THUMP and Barb lay face down, flat on the floor, not moving! No warning, no whimper, just THUMP!

I'm afraid to read further, but I can't read fast enough, desperately searching for key words such as *breathing* or *hospital*. Finally, I inhale, and go back to the THUMP.

> One student ran to get the owner of the studio who was sitting in her office working on the computer. Another student called 911. There was a fire station just down the street, so paramedics were at the studio in minutes.
>
> A third student ran down the stairs to guide the paramedics into the building and up the stairs.
>
> Barb had fainted. She revived quickly, and the paramedics took her to the hospital for twenty-four hours of observation. She'd spent the whole day golfing and was exhausted and dehydrated from the heat. The stairs and the yoga were just too much. When she got the hospital bill, she joked that it was the most expensive "free" yoga class she had ever taken and even I had to laugh.

Barb returned the following week with just a small bruise on her cheek. She still laughs about it. I can only share what I heard of the story, but I enjoy Barb's version again and again because it brings us joy.

So, when struggles come up we have our laughter that has filled our cup of energy, and we're able to give from our overflow. We're able to support ourselves and each other from our abundance.

Barb's friend, Gloria, finds herself temporarily depressed.

Usually optimistic, but that is ebbing. Although, most days, I hear her laughter before she enters the studio, but today she trudges up the stairs, not laughing. In fact, hardly speaking.

It's Barb's fifty-sixth birthday and she has decided to spend it with us.

"This is the place that I choose to be," she explains. She lost her husband to cancer not too many birthdays ago, and community, joy, and laughter are the birthday gifts she wants.

I whisper to Barb, "What's up with Gloria?"

She shakes her head.

Finally, as gently as I can, I ask Gloria. "What's wrong?"

We're a fairly frank group, so I don't feel that the question is intrusive.

Gloria responds with equal frankness, "I'm feeling pretty low. I've lost my optimism."

She walks over to the area of the room where she likes to practice and unrolls her mat. Barb unrolls her own mat next to Gloria's. I hear quiet whispers.

More students are entering the studio. As I greet each one, I notice a lovely golden glow on their faces. The soft amber hues of the sun are being reflected from the metallic building across the alley and bouncing through the studio windows. The students are also taking note of this new but temporary light that is warming our space.

Gloria seems to notice, too.

I always begin sessions with a thought or a poem. Tonight's is about seeing and celebrating the beauty of life that exists all around us. The reflected sunlight is changing rapidly as the sun drops quickly below the horizon. The poem and the sun's descent are almost simultaneous.

We begin our practice.

At the end of class, I ask Gloria to notice sunsets. Although the moon has risen during our practice, Gloria's face is glowing.

The sparkle is back. I see optimism in her eyes again and I hope it will last the week. Instead of having the fear stand in front of you and hold you back, have the fear stand behind you and push you forward.

I have found a poem called, *Collect Your Blessings* in honor of Barb's birthday and read it aloud at the class's end.

Take notice of the flowers surviving the graveled soil,

the leaf clinging to its branch in the wind,

the care extended when the kindness of strangers is witnessed . . .

Barb thanks me for a lovely birthday celebration. I tell her that she is the gift to the class, and I welcome her gratitude with open arms and heart.

This gathering of lives brings a glow to all of us for precious moments at a time, a moment no longer than the changing color of a sunset.

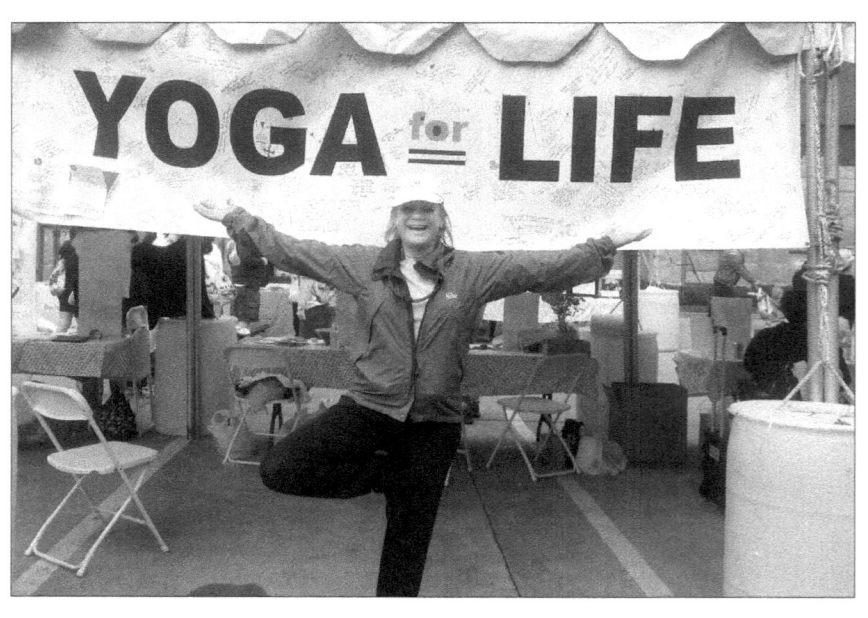

Fund-Raising

*We should cultivate the ability to say no to activities for which
we have no time, no talent, and which we have no interest or
real concern. If we learn to say no to many things, then
we will be able to say yes to things that matter most.*

—Roy Blauss

I have coordinated my students to help me this week—an eight-day yoga schedule with more than fifty classes. Half of these volunteers are people who are actively going through treatment.

The American Cancer Society flew me to Washington, D.C., for *Lobby Day* in September 2005. I was part of a group of about three hundred, all of us prepared to meet with our state representatives and senators to express our concerns over state laws and funding that does not allow screenings or treatment to those without insurance.

I was still in the middle of my own treatment and for a schoolteacher, this timing was the worst. But my students and their parents all understood, and Michael stayed home to take care of our children.

As I got on the plane, I reminded myself that this whole cancer adventure had not allowed me any leisure, rest, or disengagement.

It was always go-go-go and telling people why it's important that I go-go-go. I found my seat on the plane and plopped my laptop on the vacant seat next to mine. My hat fell off my hairless head and drew glances from people who quickly looked away. It's no longer of significance to me. I replaced it. In some ways, I wore it for them, not for me.

Three delegates represented Utah. Coincidentally, we were all marathon runners. John, a prostate and colon cancer survivor, was training for the St. George marathon and would run before and after our meetings.

I had just completed the Salt Lake City marathon and enjoyed a good jog around the district before our lobbying responsibilities began.

But it was our third delegate, Iris, who was the most impressive. I met her in the hotel lobby prior to the gathering in the dining hall for delegates from all fifty states. Hurricane Katrina had just come ashore, and we were all anxiously waiting to hear from the Gulf State delegates.

Iris is an amazing woman. She has run more than sixty marathons, one even in Antarctica. And although her age equaled the number of marathons she had ran, she was a feisty woman who doesn't act her age.

Thank goodness!

We had scheduled twenty-minute appointments with each of our state senators and representatives, but we didn't see them all. Senators Orrin Hatch and Robert Bennett sent their aides to the scheduled meeting. Congressmen Chris Cannon, Jim Matheson, and Rob Bishop met with us in person. Although Congressman Bishop could barely keep his eyes open, at least he listened to what we had traveled across the country to say.

But it was Jim Matheson who was the most receptive and responsive to hearing our requests. He even asked us if we would take a photo with him!

Fund-Raising

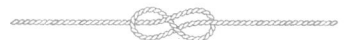

That same autumn, I decided to take my fourth-grade students to a local American Cancer Society fund-raiser. Four of them twenty percent, have been directly affected by a parent or a grandparent who has had breast cancer.

The odds are too high. I stir uneasily, seeing a nightmarish epidemic. Contributing, however, rather than lamenting helps us feel better. We're a small but mighty group of under-five-footers but bottle our energy and you could charge the planet. They run everywhere. Our fund-raiser today is a five-mile walk around Liberty Park. My only instruction, as they run to their morning responsibility, their water station is, "Don't run over anyone."

They look at me quizzically.

"What is Mrs. Conn talking about now?"

The fact is, they don't see their own motion. They hop over picnic tables, leap-frog recycling cans, circle hundred-year-old pines until they've worn moat like trenches around them. They're just being the kid inside.

I'm also trying to teach them something more abstract. "Raise your awareness, especially of your surroundings."

If they aren't aware of their own bodies flying over the picnic tables, how can they be aware of the muscles moving their bodies, the breath powering them, the connection between that picnic table and the pine tree?

Realizing the effects of cancer on the body was, indeed, raised this particular morning for Benjamin, my very own fourth grader, as well as my other twenty-one fourth-grade students. Three of them joined me on stage to warm up the crowd with some yoga exercises.

We breathed in and out, then growled through our Warrior Ones and Warrior Twos. "Ahhhhhhh," preceded my proclamation, "Warrior One!"

In unison, five thousand survivors and families draw from their gut, "Ahhhhhhh."

They are announcing their presence to the universe and to God: "We're here. We're alive. It's early on a drizzly Saturday morning. Don't mess with us."

It was fantastic.

Iris was growling, too.

I think our messages are being heard. I mean, how could you possibly avoid that much growling?

We raised fifteen hundred (1,500) dollars in three weeks for the American Cancer Society. Every penny earned was raising awareness within my students, in addition collecting money for a worthy cause.

I'm a schoolteacher. Educating kids is what it is all about for me.

The following year, September 19–20, 2006, the American Cancer Society sent me back to D.C. as an ambassador for a much larger event. Nearly four thousand (4,000) survivors from every legislative district joined me in the second semi-annual 'Celebration on the Hill'. It was a grassroots appeal to our country's lawmakers to present a personal face to cancer.

Once again, I found it an opportunity to impress upon my state's congressmen and senators, no matter how sleepy they might be, my thoughts and desires about passing laws to provide mammogram screenings for uninsured women. This particular D.C. trip also gave Michael and me the opportunity to educate our own children. We arranged for their absence from school, and we toured our nation's capital. Still adorned with "chemo curls, I reflected with amazement on the abundance of supporters. Four thousand of us are here today, each filled with hope and the desire to live out our life as we choose.

The National Mall featured a scaffold four hundred (400) feet

Fund-Raising

long and twenty (20) feet high with banners from each state promoting the "Relay for Life" fund-raiser. Each banner represented countless stories and signatures of people struggling to survive cancer.

The structure was called the "Wall of Hope." My own yoga fund-raising efforts presented twenty thousand (20,000) dollars to the American Cancer Society's Cancer Action Network along with our own banner, "Yoga for Life."

I hung it in the Utah tent on the National Mall and took photos of people standing in the Tree pose who visited our tent. It was our Tent of Hope. Hanging this labyrinth of banners took two weeks. Once it was completed, it was easy to spend hours reading, walking, and then reading and walking some more.

Nestled in the center of the maze was a searchlight four feet in diameter, aimed skyward. On the night of September 20th, the beam of light was so powerful and bright that it became a directional beacon for our family as we toured monuments throughout the district. The light represented us, and we felt a part of why it was shining for everyone to see.

This display was considered a historic event. Even government celebrities like Hillary Clinton, Newt Gingrich, and Barack Obama came out to speak to our group of survivors. I felt honored to be part of this process and to have our children be a part of it with us. When it came time for the march of silence around the reflection pool, we lit the luminaries representing cancer survivors and honoring those who had been lost. Thousands encircled the reflection pool. When we looked back toward the people who marched behind us and ahead to those marching in front, we realized that the ends met. We could not tell where we began nor where we ended.

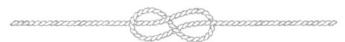

Two years after my first lobbying visit, almost to the day in 2007, I read a feature article about Iris. Her breast cancer had metastasized after almost ten years of dormancy. The reporter quoted her, "God better help me change my attitude because I'm not gonna be much fun up there with him if he doesn't."

The recurrence had been discovered during a check-up prior to a Lance Armstrong hundred-mile bike ride fundraiser, she told me when I telephoned her. I can tell she is really pissed off, but she is still wanting to go-go-go!

Holding Open the Space

When we face the worst that can happen in any situation, we grow. When circumstances are at their worst, we can find our best.
—ELaurenbeth Kubler-Ross

Judd emailed me today. He has worked very hard with our fund-raiser, showing up when his ANC was low—well below five hundred (500). (Absolute Neutrophil Count, a measure of white blood cells that resist infections. The normal is 1.5 to 8.0 (1,500 to 8,000/mm3).

Judd's doctors were concerned, speculating about what may be causing the drop.

We both knew that his white blood cells were too low, signaling severe neutropenia and placing him at a high risk of infection. He came to the studio to help me raise money for cancer, but I think Judd was available and present for reasons far exceeding that day's purpose. Judd is young and handsome. He has many supportive friends and comes from a large family, many of whom I've been fortunate enough to meet. Judd wasn't at the studio because of our fundraising event or because of me. He continued to show up to class after class after class, relaying the message of hope because this is what he was living on, the possibility that he would be well again.

He's feeling badly, but he continues come to the studio for our *Yoga for Life* campaign. He tells his story to groups of people who practice yoga, then returns to the lobby in hopes that they will donate to the American Cancer Society at the table he staffs. He hopes they will raise money for cancer research, specifically to fund an organization that will lobby for changes in our current laws that include mammogram screening for uninsured women.

Today is Judd's birthday. A group of friends are sending him back to New York City, his former home, for a week of excitement and freedom from concern. Revisiting a familiar place reminds him of a time of no restraint—a time before leukemia.

He told me that, after his return to Salt Lake City, he will move to Hawaii. It is a place that nurtures his soul, his mind, and his body simultaneously. He has found another community.

He wrote, expressing gratitude for the A Quality Life Community class. I remind him that he creates the class by his attendance and all that he brings with him. I simply hold the space open so it can take place.

I open my dictionary to Yoga: *Union, yoking with the Supreme Spirit*. I flip back to the F's and look up Friendship: *Aptness to unite; affinity; harmony*.

Letting Go of Pain

A true friend stabs you in the front.
—Oscar Wilde

Releasing a painful past is difficult, especially since the event causing the pain had so significantly defined us for a short but intense period. In releasing the pain, do we release the event altogether? Does releasing the pain deny that the event occurred? Is it time to begin redefining ourselves?

I ask these questions using plural pronouns as I cannot separate my individual struggle, yes, pain, from my family's struggle, in whatever ways it manifested but, in the end, pain.

In August 2008, in celebration of three friends who turned fifty, a group of fourteen people took a one-week cruise up Alaska's inside passage. Four amongst us were teenagers, one of whom turned fifteen at sea. The trip marked the first time Michael and I had traveled together without our children since their births. It took careful consideration, coordination, and collaboration. It was significant.

These people are my *Big Chill* group, the name coming from the 1983 movie. Aboard ship we were once again that group of young men and women living in the Haight-Ashbury, Noe Valley, and Castro District of San Francisco in the first half of the 1980s. Our past took place in the midst of an AIDS epidemic, struggles with graduate school, lovers with all preferences of lifestyles, seeking careers and the individual paths that would later define us—or, at least, would define us for a moment of time. We have managed to keep in touch with each other through marriages, lovers, childbirths, and adoptions. We try to see each other once a year and succeed about fifty percent of the time. But this trip required one hundred percent participation. We did it, and we were grateful for the week we spent at sea with each other.

The days were filled with adventures. We all went off the boat in different directions. Ocean kayaking, cycling to blue glaciers, dog sledding, helicopter rides, train rides to sites that Jack London had used as settings for his stories. Between the fourteen of us, we covered a lot of ground.

Our group dinners every night at 8:00 PM celebrated the events of the day, and our adult table of ten was always the last to leave so the tolerant wait staff could clear it. The volume of our laughter consistently exceeded acceptable decibel levels, but not once were we reprimanded. It was the time spent around the table that meant the most to me. These friends had supported Michael and me through our cancer adventure.

When it came time to sign up for the *On Deck for the Cure* walk around the ship, we all walked or ran at our own pace. With whales swimming off our port bow in the still, blue-gray waters, I could think of no better place to let go of my pain. In releasing remnants of whatever I held onto from the past three-plus years, I gained more in love and faith of these sustained friendships. It was this group who showed me, "We'll share your pain until you feel it no longer." And they did.

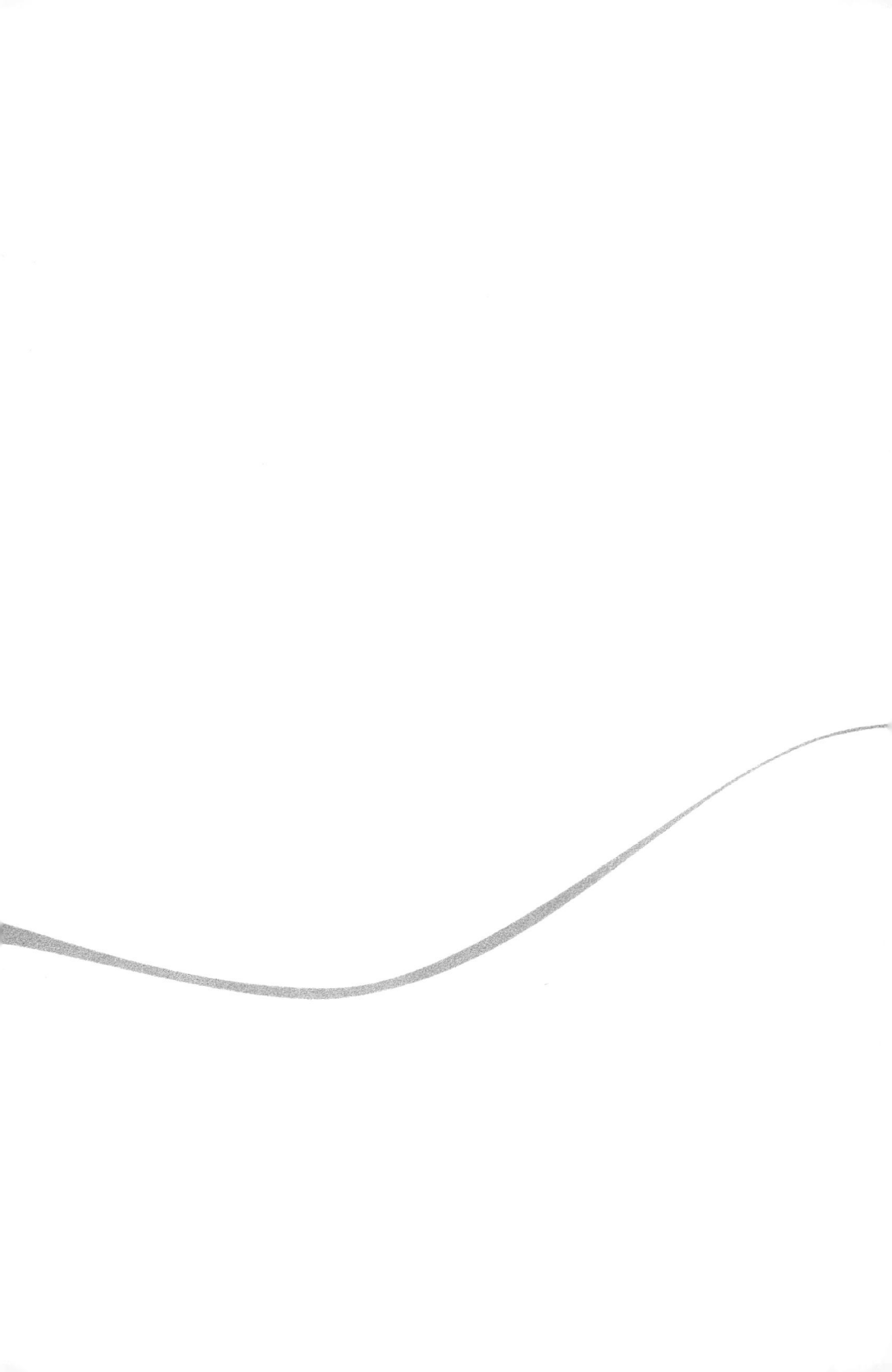

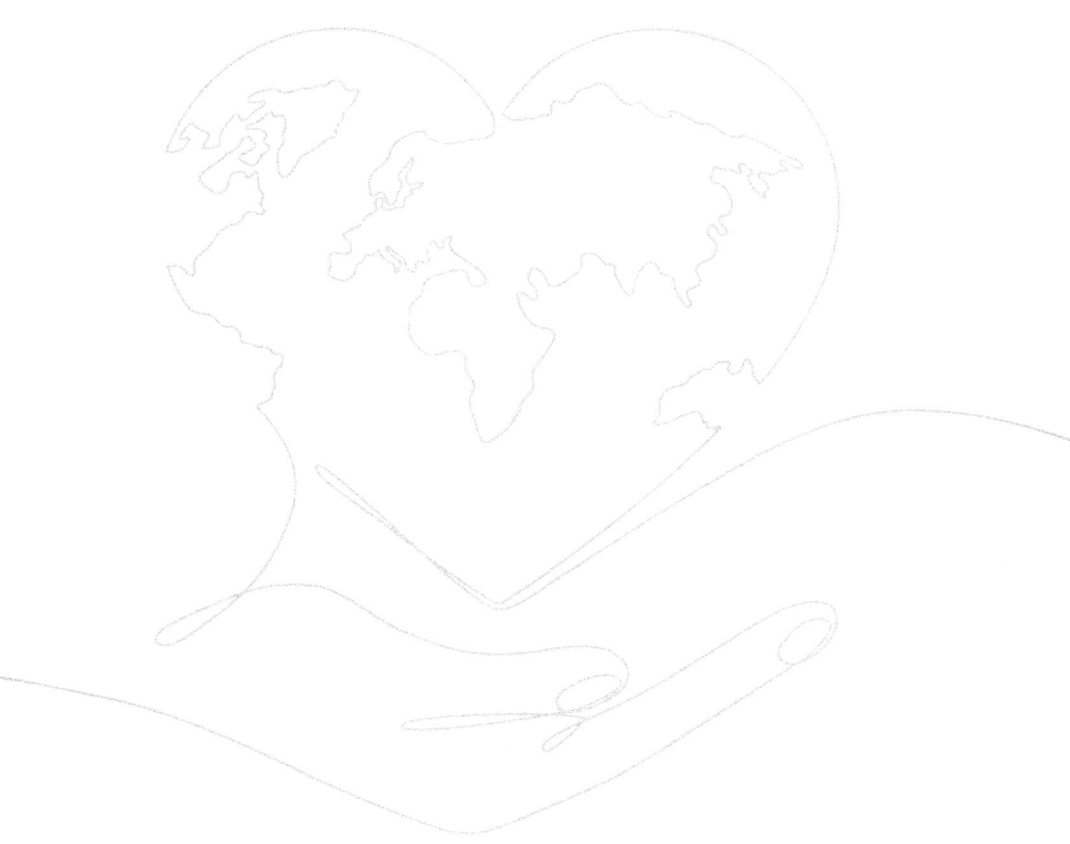

PART FOUR
My World

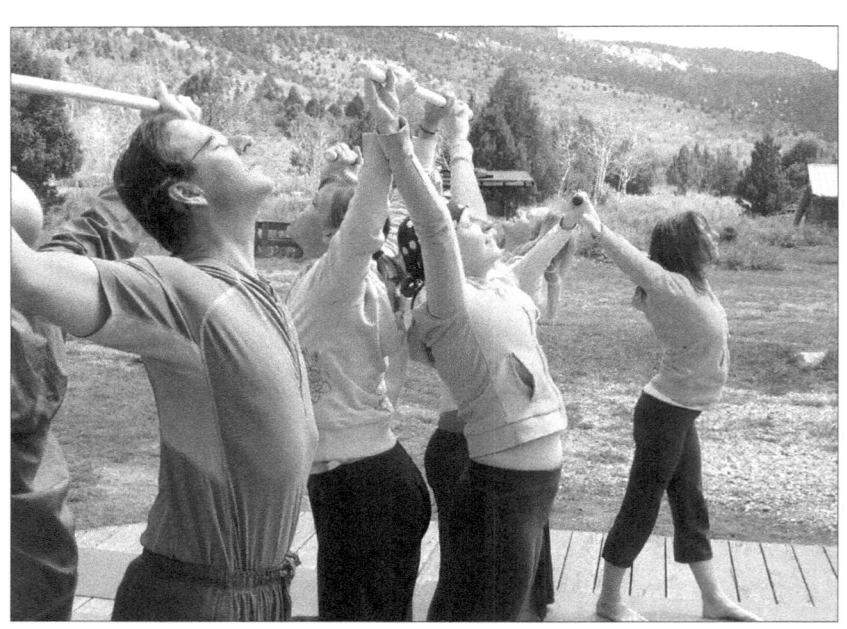

My Dream of Yoga

Who are we, not to shine?
—Marianne Williamson

My dream of yoga was to continue to teach my weekly A Quality Life Community class for survivors, caregivers, and loved ones; continue taking survivors and their families on mountain retreats; and later, a home where families could stay while their parent or child receives hospital treatments. This home would act as *mini retreats*, same accouterments, just near the hospital. The class would be free. Remember, *Bringing Wellness to Life*.

Yoga is much more than physical. The Yoga Sutras are an ancient collection of aphorisms that established the practice of yoga. In Sanskrit, *sutra* means literally a rope or thread that holds things together. In the second century, Patanjali, the author and founder of the system of yoga, wrote them down. Although there exists some debate about the authorship of these sutras, Patanjali is a revered name in the yoga tradition. He is considered to be one of the most famous Sanskrit grammarians of ancient India. The sage Patanjali defines yoga as chitta vritti nirodha. Chitta is the consciousness which includes the mind, the intellect, and the ego. Yoga is a method of silencing the vibrations of the chitta.

Though brief, the Yoga sutras are an enormously influential work on yoga philosophy and practice, held by principal proponents of yoga such as B. K. S. Iyengar. Iyengar (Guruji) is a ninety-year-old living legend who has studied and practiced yoga since age sixteen when he met his own guru, Sri T. Krishnamacharya. His style of teaching yoga is called Iyengar yoga and is now being followed by certified teachers across the world. Iyengar states, "When I practice, I am a philosopher. When I teach, I am a scientist. When I demonstrate, I am an artist.

In these Yoga sutras, Patanjali prescribes adherence to the eight *limbs,* or spokes in a wagon wheel to quiet one's mind. With the rising popularity of yoga classes, the teacher may mention these sutras as part of his or her instruction but may not teach them systematically or work with students on practicing them. But in my survivor class, these limbs are essential—synonymous with life and living that life.

My friends, Rolf and Mariam Gates, have generously contributed two hundred copies of *Meditations from the Mat* (New York: Anchor, 2002) to my A Quality Life Community class. I give a copy to each new student so that he or she will have a take-home guide for understanding the yoga sutras. The book is written like a daily journal—three hundred and sixty-five messages describing each aspect of the Patanjali's yoga path. Rolf and his co-author, Katrina Kenison, describe each path in a way that makes the concept easy for a non-yogi to absorb, and the feedback from my students is that this is the book they keep on their nightstands.

For example, in *Meditations from the Mat*, Rolf and Katrina write, "The final aspect of the yoga path is isvara-pranidhana or surrender to God. Faith, surrender, devotion. Faith in what? Surrender to what? Devotion to what?"

The answers to these questions cannot be found in any book; they are inscribed in our hearts. In my Anusara yoga practice we are taught that everything we need to be complete is within us—right at this very moment. It is simply a matter of being able to recognize it. We don't need to be yoginis already to begin the process of healing ourselves.

On the nights that our class meets, we begin with the first principle of Anusara Yoga: *Open to Grace.* In this principle, we open our hearts to welcome all the beauty around us. Here is where our evening practice begins. It is the foundation of our movement, no matter how soft or how active, no matter how subtle or insistent.

Marianne Williamson reminds us clearly, "Our deepest fear is not that we are inadequate. Our deepest fear is that we are powerful beyond measure."

At the end of class, I tell the students to lie on their mats in Savasana, the final resting pose. I take each student's head between my hands and, as Kim did for me, cradle it so that he or she can release. Faith, surrender, devotion. As Ms. Williamson concludes, "And as we let our own light shine, we unconsciously give other people permission to do the same. As we are liberated from our own fear, our presence automatically liberates others."

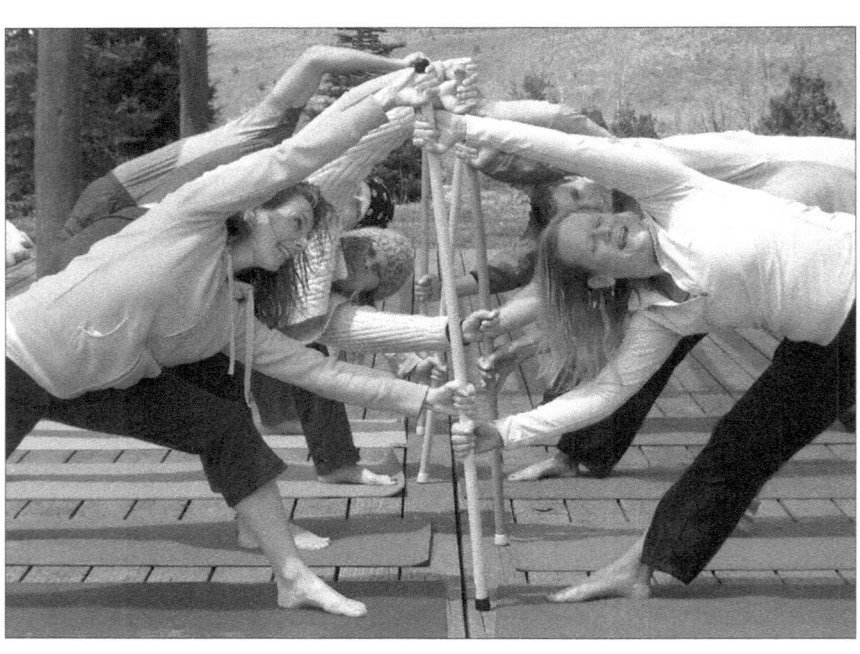

Women Beyond Cancer

*"A journey into how mind, body and spirit are inseparable;
We are hard-wired for Bliss"*

—Dr. Candace Pert

"I have another community."

Michael was doing the dishes, and he took a deep breath.

Is he rolling his eyes?

He sighed. "Which one is it now?"

He knows me all too well and realizes that the futility of struggling against my desire to be inclusive.

I cradle his face in my hands and squeeze his cheeks together, pursing out his lips for that *chubby baby* expression. I kiss him, slowly and thoroughly, then take a step back.

"Well, it's actually a sub-community under the guise of larger community."

His eyes look tired. After the dishes, our kids are waiting for him upstairs to play *tickle-monster*.

I suspect he's thinking, 'How much time is this one going to cost me?'

My A Quality Life Community class had now formed a core of regulars who help each other as much as I have helped them. This sub-community is unintentionally exclusive in its inclusiveness.

We rely on each other and supporting one another outside the studio. We are bound to each other by a common illness, but it is our *wellness* that nourishes us.

Women Beyond Cancer is a non-profit organization that serves the emotional, physical, and spiritual needs of women with any type of cancer. They emphasize not just surviving but living beyond it.

"We're Cancer thrivers!" our Q of Lifers proclaim.

Ten women from my class accepted the invitation of Women Beyond Cancer to a free retreat in a beautiful home resort in the nearby mountains. I had asked the director to be one of the group, not the yoga instructor. It was a conscious decision to pay attention to my own needs.

We gathered to share continuing stories of life with and without cancer in the amber glow from a huge stone fireplace. The hearth warmed our bodies from the outside, and the conversation warmed us from the inside.

We already knew each other, but saying, "My biggest fear is that I will die from this." It never gets easier.

Carrie has been part of our program since its inception. She is a wife, a mother of two young children, and oh yeah—she's a cancer survivor. She is also an infectious disease pediatric specialist, a wealth of terrifying information at her fingertips. I don't know how she manages to let her children leave the house to face our contagious, germ-infested world but she does.

I smiled. "Ignorance is bliss."

Carrie told us about her first *Race for the Cure* experience.

"I'm not a runner. I exercise, but I don't really run." Somehow, she and her seven-year-old son got in the crowd of runners and were being encouraged to, "move on up, move on up."

"I was in the middle of treatment. My bald head and grip on my child's hand pretty much told the whole story."

Before she knew it, she was *encouraged* right up to the front starting line in the group of seeded runners who not only planned on running the entire race but planned on winning it as well.

"Um, I'm not a runner. I'm not a runner," she called out, but apparently no one was listening.

Everyone was too focused on beginning this race.

Suddenly the starter's gun sounded. "And they're off!" the race director announced.

"I squeezed my son's hand, and we ran for our lives! The runners continued to push us. We ran faster than we ever have before. "But I'm not a runner! I'm not!"

"Still, no one seemed to hear me."

By the time they reached the first mile marker, the clock read *seven minutes*. These two non-runners ran a seven-minute mile in their very first race!

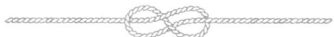

Mare, short for Marilyn, our over-energized leader from Women Beyond Cancer, took us on a three-hour snowshoeing adventure. The snow was deep and glistened on the aspen tree branches when the morning sun hit them.

"Gorgeous! If ever I dreamed of a place where we could be together outside of the yoga studio, this would be the place." I was filled with joy as I gazed upon our group, poised against the backdrop of the pines.

We stood on the side of a mountain and Mare led us to a snow-covered meadow surrounded by trees. To the south the peak loomed overhead and the valley floor lay to the north. The air was crisp, our noses cold to the touch; but our bodies were warm, and our hearts were filled with adrenaline and love.

"Where are we going now?" one of the women asked nervously.

I snicker. I love hiking alone or with my dog. I forgot that being outside without a sidewalk in sight may not be the norm for some.

When I was younger, I led groups of troubled kids into the wilderness for days at a time. People often asked, "Aren't you afraid they will run away from you?" My response was always the same, "The wilderness terrifies most people. Being alone in the woods would be their biggest fear."

Lovely Mare asked us to make our own path. She was instantly met with resistance.

"What do you mean—our own path?"

But Mare just smiled. "Trust me."

We snowshoed into the trees halfway up our mountain in ten different directions. The trees masked the sound of the other nine but amplified the sounds of nature on my own path, the animals and the birds, and the restful, peaceful sounds of quiet.

The trees protected each of us. We trusted them. The blue sky, snow, mountain, meadow, woods—solitude—the combination provided a balance to the chaos that brought us here, equilibrium for the world that awaits us down in the valley.

I surrendered to the power of silence and the harmony of nature before my eyes. I remembered that I am part of this harmony, not separated from it. I don't have to fight this movement. Resistance only encouraged more resistance. I became the silence.

When we all returned to the meadow, it was as if we had all received the same memo, *Move with the flow—we are the flow.*

Snowshoe yoga. You don't know if you can do it unless you try.

We bend forward and twist our bodies, with our huge platformed snowshoes, we form a bond with our inner circle of friends. We reach to the sky as a symbol of higher consciousness. We open our bodies and our minds to be receptive to our world. We long to live so that we may live longer.

Michael has taught me, "If I surrender and trust that this is what I truly desire, then and only then, will I be available to receive what I truly need."

Laughter promotes laughter. Love promotes love. Internally, there is no difference.

Dr. Candace Pert, a neuroscientist who discovered the cellular bonding site for endorphins in the brain states, "Supporting the soul by cradling it promotes the growth of healthy cells. When we smile, laugh, and love, our body responds with a cascade of events that promote only health."

In Dr. Pert's book, *Everything You Need to Know to Feel Go(o)d*, (Hayhouse, 2007), she writes, "We know that our body heals with prayer. We know we feel better when we're in a loving environment. When people support one another, we can venture farther down the path of recovery. The mind, body, and spirit are inseparable; we are hard-wired for bliss, which is both physical and divine."

Our beautiful meadow is like the eye of a hurricane, calm, serene, beautiful. The challenge lay at the meadow's periphery where trees led to steeper peaks. It crests turbulently, in unsettled snow.

The tree line, our destination, opened up to bluer skies; and we were drawn to meet this edge. We stood above the valley and felt the glory of being on top of our world.

Then Mare asked, "Can you make it to the peak?"

We chorused, "Yes!"

Some of the women had never put on snowshoes in their lives. For others, they had, but it had been years. But it didn't matter. Our trek to the top took three hours. By the time we were home again, we were hungry, but we could hardly contain our excitement. With each step, our cancer, however we defined it, was being conquered. Had we stopped before attaining the peak it somehow represented defeat or giving in.

Not today!

The retreat was our sanctuary. We were a diverse group of women. We wore many different hats and many titles. We were physicians, teachers, accountants, massage therapists, architects, counselors, biologists, mothers, wives, and lovers.

Friends.

We were all friends.

We were all absolutely brilliant women. There was not one among us who didn't share a story about the powers of healing. The retreat took on a tone of a healing workshop.

Erin is a biochemist and taught my A Quality Life Community class while I was in Australia. When she was not in her lab, she was in the yoga studio.

She asked, "What if we were to believe that we could heal ourselves? What if this belief was a common one, never subjected to disbelief?"

She tells us about a five-year old boy with cystic fibrosis. This child, has had no inflammation events or hospitalizations since birth.

Erin poised a question. "What if the environment of the cell could be altered by something we cause? The cell within the cell wall—the interior environment and its exterior—could change. What if we can influence that change?"

There was a long pause while we processed the idea.

For Dr. Pert, the mind is not just in the brain—it is also in the body.

"The vehicle that the mind and body use to communicate with each other is the chemistry of emotion." The chemicals in question are molecules, short chains of amino acids called peptides and receptors, that she believes to be the *biochemical correlate of emotion.*

"The peptides can be found in your brain, but also in your stomach, your muscles, your glands and all your major organs, sending messages back and forth."

After decades of research, Dr. Pert is finally able to make clear how *emotion creates the bridge between mind and body.*

Our bodies have natural body triggers. "For example, *the fight or flight trigger*," Erin explained. We calm our bodies through breathing techniques, allowing our minds to process information without the panic."

I once had an allergic reaction to Taxol, a chemotherapy modality, and I used breathing to still my body's terror at the poison's invasion. Understanding calmness on a cellular level may encourage our doctors to be more empathic to patients' requests to be treated on other levels than just the medical one.

"What if we could practice influencing the environment of the cell in such a way that it

changes it completely, thus, changing our life?"

Erin paused and looked around the room at all of our faces.

We are rapt.

Dr. Pert explains in her book that, "Perception and awareness play a vital part in health and longevity."

We understand that the secret of cancer is to not feed it or give it any recognition beyond what is necessary. Rather, the secret is to love the working, healthy parts of our bodies—love the parts that are nourishing us.

Self-acceptance begins with just that—the self.

"Which comes first, the mind or chemistry?" asked Dr. Pert, "It is the crux of the difference between Eastern and Western thought. In Eastern, the consciousness precedes reality. In Western, we think consciousness is a secretion of the brain, like urine is a secretion of the kidneys."

As our group of women continued to contemplate and discuss these thoughts, I continue to read aloud, "There is a very close correspondence between the highest, most concentrated areas of enrichment of a certain neuropeptides and where the chakras are classically supposed to be—the eastern system of seven energy center."

Do we treat physical conditions from an emotional point of

view or vice versa? The answer is you simultaneously do both, because they're flip sides of the same thing. The key word is balance.

The conversation continues, drifting toward areas of our lives that feel unfulfilled. Could this be our illness? In reality, has cancer just tapped us on the shoulder, getting our attention so that we can give it to these other areas of our lives? That was true for me. Cancer made things clearer, brighter, simpler. It woke me up.

What areas of our lives are we turning away from? The doctor in our group is highly respected, her walls thick with awards and recognition certificates, yet she retreats from this demonstrated esteem and affection. The stay-at-home mother in our group expresses disorganization in all aspects of her life—mentally, physically, and familial.

She struggles to release the clutter. What is it symbolizing? The writer in our group cycles uneasily between her fear of writing and her desire to trust her impulse to write. She resists being identified in photographs. She pauses long over signing waivers, even the one allowing her to participate in this retreat; yet she knows that remaining invisible conflicts with her belief that she must be accountable for her life.

Carrie tells us about rafting on the Colorado River. This is an activity she could never do before cancer because she was much too fearful of the waves and the current. The *what-ifs* would storm her imagination with rafts being flipped, her children sailing through the air. She always opted out when her family suggested a river trip vacation.

After cancer, she was the one to ask, "Should we raft down the Colorado?"

Her family rejoiced at her newfound strength and bravery! She backpedaled, but only a little. "Now, not a class five rapid. Maybe class three. Well…maybe class four. This is our first trip. Let's not get carried away!"

I know how much suffering is in this room, and I ask myself, *Why isn't there more sadness? I hear only laughter.*

A previous WBC survivor had crocheted a pair of large breasts with a gorgeous set of nipples, then sewed them on a crocheted band that wrapped around the chest. The fortunate wearer appears to be quite endowed. We passed it around at the dinner table. Every one of us wanted to try it on. We all wanted photos of ourselves with breasts again.

We finished the meal with waves of laughter, then started telling stories of never having to wear a bra again, of choosing our preferred breast-size. This was the *woman* part of *women beyond cancer*. We dealt with the with the same hot flashes, sore joints, bone density tests, menopause before age forty-five, and total lack of a sex drive.

"Don't get me started on vaginal dryness," one of the women shouts.

"Ahhhh, yes!" We could all agree.

Within a year of weaning Abigail, I was told that I was peri menopausal. Now I'm living on the other end of the menopause spectrum, transported quickly due to my cancer adventure.

Anecdotes of raising fourth graders in our forties, husbands' socks and holey underwear. It never really mattered if a particular storyline came to a neat conclusion. Someone always had a contribution to make to this particular theme.

More laughter.

Locker-room satire. Our children are too young to manage their ice hockey uniforms alone but too old to have any of their peers witness Mom assisting them. "Well, then, why am I here? The odor alone, honey, is killing me!"

We're sitting in a room filled with love, with laughter, tears in our eyes, bellies aching, and our sorrows weakened.

Our bodies have brought us this laughter drawn from underarms and underwear, unleashing our playfulness remembered from years ago. The sadness dissipates, and the belief in magic returns. All things are possible. We hold hope in our cupped palms. Love surrounds our hearts and pumps through our veins. We are now feeling more well than ill, more alive than sick— essentially, just *feeling* more.

Sundance Yoga Retreat

*When one tugs at a single thing in nature,
he finds it attached to the rest of the world.*
—John Muir

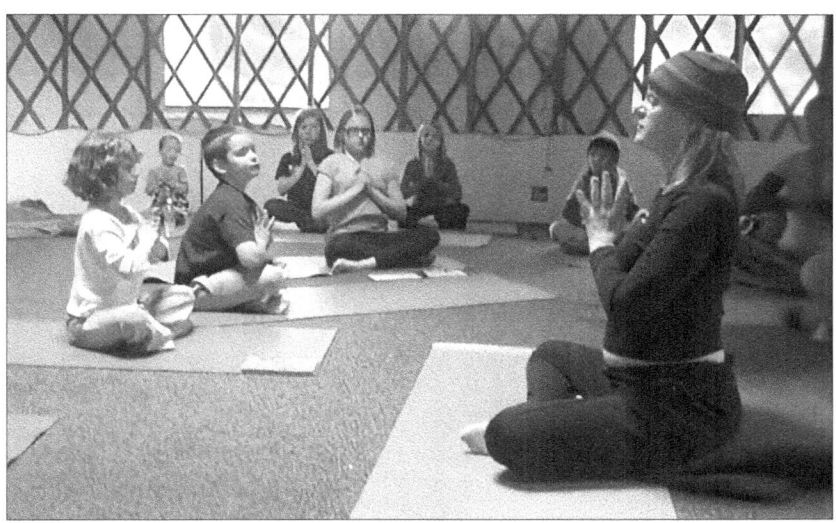

Eighteen months of fundraising and planning has led us to this point. I find myself standing in the parking lot at the Sundance Resort with the sound of nothing but rushing water. Nestled at the base of twelve-thousand-foot Mount Timpanogos in Utah, the Sundance Resort calls the Sundance Preserve its home.

We arrive exhausted and exuberant at the same time. Over the course of four days, my friend Zach will teach and practice yoga with cancer survivors and their mates, and I will teach and practice with the children of those survivors. We are playful, hopeful, and determined. We're here to learn from one another.

In our retreat, we have specific groups intermingled with those who simply want to practice. These groups have largely been funded by businesses in Salt Lake City, Utah and my friends and family. I was able to meet with CEO's of companies who agreed to make large contributions; everyone else gave in increments of twenty-dollar bills.

I had an emotional moment opening up an envelope from a twelve-year-old child from Iran who gave twelve dollars, one for every year of their life. Eight thousand dollars was raised to bring together individuals and families who have experienced a traumatic episode in their life, whether cancer or divorce, we come as hopeful beings seeking a healing opportunity.

Twelve of the thirteen children, ages four to eleven years, have experienced an upheaval in their life, temporarily turning it upside down. It is my job this long weekend to try and right this situation, even if only for a moment.

The adults have a larger range of vibrancy. They arrive with the expectation of reprieve. Healthy individuals intermingle with those currently going through a protocol of chemotherapy. Participants are single, married, or divorced, many of them are parents.

In reference to the overall design of creating such a reprieve, Sundance is considered.

"This place in the mountains, amid nature's casualness toward death and birth, is the perfect host for the inspiration of ideas, harsh at times, life threatening in its winters

of destruction, but tender in attention to the details of every petal of every wildflower resurrected in the spring. Nature and creativity obey the same laws, to the same end, life."

— Robert Redford.

Nature represented itself well throughout the four days. When we arrive, the temperature hovered in the high seventies. By Friday, rain threatened, and clouds insulated the humidity.

Saturday the air turned cooler and thicker, the rain came, and kept us inside all day. We were leaving Sunday and woke up to snow. Large winter flakes fell and stuck to the ground. Each twig on every tree was coated with snow, winter announced itself, even if for just a moment.

Later in the day when the retreat came to an end, the air had warmed up and the clouds dissipated. The sky opened and the sun's rays touched the ground, kissed our cheeks, and brought smiles to our faces. We had accomplished the work we set out to do.

The following day was Monday, and I had an appointment with Rose, my massage therapist. I described the weather patterns of each day, and she observed, "Honey, that's because each person was diagnosed with cancer during a different season. The magic lies within the retreat offering. Each day represented a different season to help bring each survivor back to their beginnings of their diagnosis."

Sundance is a place of shared community, art, recreation, and people who appreciate the beauty of nature and desire to preserve it. But it is also a place for the community to meet and, in our case through the practice of yoga, and the practice of play, we meet to build our dreams.

One four-year-old describes her mom's elation when she arrived at their Sundance home. "She raised her hands and jumped up and down. We made it!"

Her eleven-year-old sister described with more detail, that since their mom's diagnosis over two years ago, they hadn't really seen her show such enthusiasm.

This was my dream. To have people embrace themselves with the returned hope that a cancer experience didn't actually take anything away, but rather added a dimension to our lives that brought us closer. At night, when all of those whom we love are fast asleep, we hold our loved one. *We're okay. We're going to make it.*

Friday represented the season of fall and the children, and I ventured out for a two-mile hike with a four-hundred-foot elevation gain to see beaver dams and a waterfall. Our nature guide is part of a donation package that Sundance provides. They donate the Yoga Yurt and the Nature Center Yurt for us to create and practice in. Robbie, our twenty-four-year-old guide, is fun, and a perfect match for our wild group. His voice, although proper in tone, expresses just the right amount of humor-frequency to be caught by an alert eight-year-old.

His mannerisms remind me more of a forty-five-year-old businessman who made eye contact with each person, shook everyone's hand, and asked for their name. But his loose clothing, hair in his eyes, and electric guitar in hand, tells me that he is in the middle of his youth, and loving every minute of it.

Prior to our hike, he prepares our group of eager beavers by singing the *Three R's* by Jack Johnson, *Reduce, Reuse, Recycle*. Unbeknownst to Robbie, Jack Johnson songs have been an on-going theme throughout my past year of teaching children back in Salt Lake City.

I particularly love the songs from the Curious George CD, *With My Own Two Hands*, a song about self and community empowerment to feel love and act responsibly has been a frequently played song over the past ten months in my kid's yoga class.

We choreographed sign language to the song and often close the yoga practice with this signing song. To hear Robbie play a song from this same album, without any prompting from me, only reaffirms that we are all right where we are supposed to be, in alignment with our intentions for this retreat.

As the children sing, "Reduce, Reuse, Recycle" in their hip popping, bottom wiggling, high voice-silly face expressions, I pack water in backpacks preparing for our hike. Litt, with her two-foot-long brown hair sways back and forth with the beat of the guitar.

In the mountains, our distractions shift from busy city life to nature. Slowing down to be more aware of silence, we begin to hear. The children and I focus on the sounds of various birds, the rapid velocity of spring run-off in the streams surrounding Sundance, the shapes of the mountains, the number of dams the local beavers have created and the number of times the water falls in Stewart Falls.

These are welcome distractions bringing energy to the eyes and bodies of my young students rather than dividing and depleting energy from them. I love watching their immediate connection to nature.

Yoga extends far beyond our yurt. Today it is on the trail. We sing, chant, and laugh much of the way. Robbie shows us plants that help the earth and plants that hurt it. He explains how nature demonstrates its own natural remedies to maintain this balance; he tells the children that the act of achieving balance is all around us, all we need to do is see it. They somehow grasp this concept immediately.

Everything is seen as a playful opportunity, and no one is asking to be entertained. The children move in harmony with nature, the way nature intended. I have read that the Sundance Preserve is dedicated to maintaining the balance of art, nature and community. I look upon my group of thirteen children demonstrating this very thing. I move the group of little yoginis into a circle in a meadow that will soon burst with beautiful wildflowers. We practice several sun salutations and resting poses. One in particular that the kids love is called *Lizard-on-a-rock*.

Seven mini falls make up Stewart Falls, and it flows into the creek, meanders down the mountain, and eventually drops into our retreat location where it winds around each cabin.

Ryan, an adorable first grader asks, "If I drop a stick into the creek now, will I see it again when we reach my cabin?"

Being a believer of *All Things Possible* I couldn't tell him no with 100% certainty. Knowing that the likelihood was remote, given the velocity of flow and the many obstacles lying in the stick's path, I also know that I have to come up with an answer that appeals to his wisdom, as well as to his sense of adventure.

So, I told him, "Let's give it a try."

We mark the stick to make it easy for us to spot, then we dropped it into the creek. We stood and watched it for as far as we could see.

"You know, our lives are like your stick. The world moves fast around us and there are many bumps in the road that slow us down. When we release the things that hold meaning, like your stick, we always want to see them again. However, if that doesn't happen, I always hope that it brings joy to the next person who it comes to just as it brought us joy.

Ryan looks up at me with these huge brown eyes and draws in a big breath. "Thank you for giving me this opportunity."

His response made me want to run down the mountain, drag his mother out of her own yoga practice to ask for a copy of his birth certificate. I needed to verify the year that he was actually born so I could then denounce its authenticity. I know thirty-five-year-olds who strive to become this wise!

"It is the mission of the Sundance Preserve to inspire action for the benefit of civil society." I snicker recalling Ryan's response,

"Yes, I think we have met this mission today!"

Mother Nature teaches us much about ourselves because so many of our own physical and emotional systems have parallels in the natural world. One need only observe the manner in which diverse elements of nature work together to form a unified ecosystem to see the merits of cooperation.

The yoga community comes from all walks of life, but one belief is shared,: our community should represent who we are and what we believe. How quickly I saw strangers become friends, new friends become close, and old friends become relatives.

A mantra that I've taught the children in my yoga classes is, The Gayatri Mantra. The Sanskrit version and one of its English translations are as follows:

AUM BHOOR BHUWAH SWAHA,
TAT SAVITUR VARENYAM
BHARGO DEVASAYA DHEEMAHI
DHIYO YO NAHA PRACHODAYAT

Everything on the Earth, in the heavens and between

Rises from one effulgent source.

If my thoughts, words, and deeds, reflected this complete understanding of unity

I would be the peace I am seeking in this moment.

– Translation by Donna Farhi

The children grasp these mantras with ease. What is more astounding, however, is that they seem to understand it completely.

When I say this aloud to my friends, my son often interjects, with a *duh!* tone in his voice, "Mom, it's because we're closer to the source!"

But we made up the simple mantra that brought us home from our hike. It was one that held much meaning for the kids and me. Our hike ended around dinnertime. Robbie informed us that the two four-year-olds were the youngest children he had taken up the four-hundred-foot elevation to the falls.

The older children were taking care of the younger ones making my job easy, but we were feeling fatigue and hunger pains. Our mantra consisted of our immediate needs and was sung in order of the events soon to follow:

Nature Shack!

Get a snack!

Mommy!

Dinner!

This mantra brought us down the mountain. Little four-year-old Justice, would only repeat one line of it, "Mommy!" She followed it with a quiet giggle.

I held her hand while we hiked, periodically carrying her.

It wasn't until three weeks later, while watching video interviews of our family participants, that I realized just how important it was to have children present at the retreat.

One woman said, "I could never truly relax on vacations or retreats when my children weren't present. I could feel my heart strings stretched from my location to theirs. Concerns over their well-being preoccupied my mind. At the retreat, my mind was at rest. My children were happy and experiencing their own yoga. Everyone was at peace. This retreat was *Just Desserts!*"

Reprieve

REPRIEVE: *to cancel or postpone;
any respite, temporary relief, or escape.*

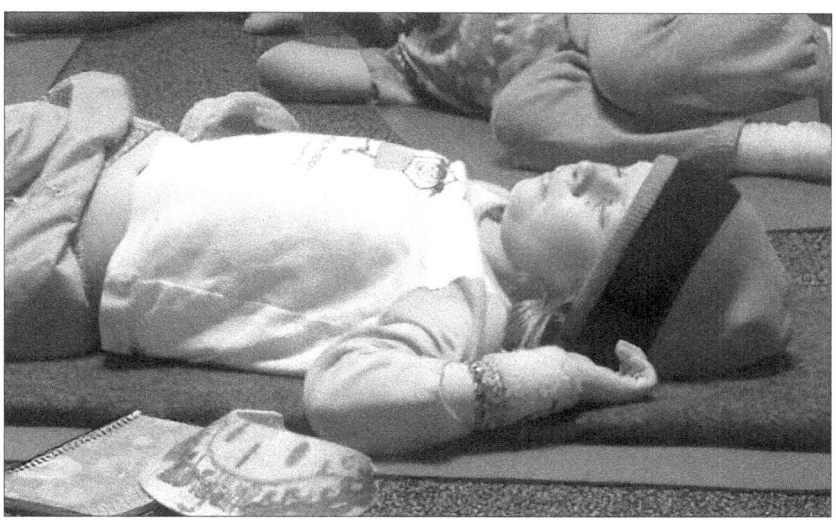

To be honest, I have felt all of these definitions during various times throughout my own cancer adventure. During times when my life was filled with needles being forced into my arm only to be met with resistance to the needle, from my body. I discovered that no amount of will, or determination could change my body's reaction. My arm simply closed down its veins.

Reprieve from pain, this is what my body was telling me.

MY cancer adventure is not really my own, I must admit. it is shared with those that I love. In addition, my cancer adventure includes other people and their own journey. It just so happens to be the thing that binds us together. Without words spoken, each of the above reprieve definitions can be discussed amongst us; even the one about *a respite from impending punishment, as from execution or a sentence of death.*

It's an elusive thought to think that my students are immune to long-term illness or to death. It is true that cancer feels better after a yoga practice and, yet, I've had to say good-bye to people that I wasn't done with.

People for whom, themselves, weren't who were not done living. People who were still raising children, and people who were happily married, and people who still longed to live. My emotions still reside just below the surface of my skin when I bring these thoughts of my friends to the forefront of my mind. My tears flow from my eyes with ease. It's this part of life and living this life that I still struggle with. These are people who shared a space and time together with me and with others like us; we are all different; and yet…we are all very similar.

No words can best describe my feelings other than, "I simply, miss them."

There are times when I practice yoga to celebrate their lives. Other times, I practice so I can support my own life. Often times, simply, I practice so I can make sense of it all.

This morning, I practiced with a woman who told me that her nephew had a rare form of cancer that if diagnosed after the child turns one-year-old, the chance of full recover lessens. Her nephew had an attentive pediatrician and was able to confirm the cancer diagnosis when he was nine months old. He is now four years old now and runs around like all other healthy children his age. He's happy and carefree. He lives his life as if completely unaffected by his cancer experience.

His mother, this woman's sister, is not as fortunate. She never processed her child's illness and therefore cannot celebrate his wellness. As odd as this may sound, her optimism surrounding her child's cancer is now keeping her from being optimistic about her child's health. She is still fighting the cancer and has not yet progressed to celebrating his wellness. She is fearful of it returning and doesn't want to be caught off guard *again*.

She's stuck.

Releasing fear and placing trust after a traumatic experience requires a tremendous amount trust in trauma-informed therapies. This trust and a properly matched therapeutic approach can bring wellness. It is my desire to see this family and others like them revisit this place trusting the therapeutic process, exploring the boundaries of its healing capacity. It is my belief that it is in this place of release that true healing and life begins anew.

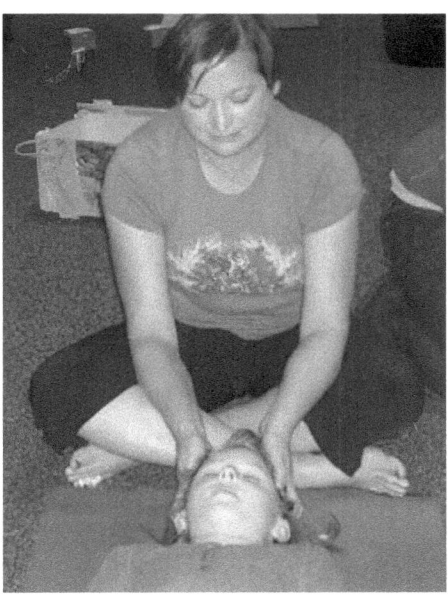

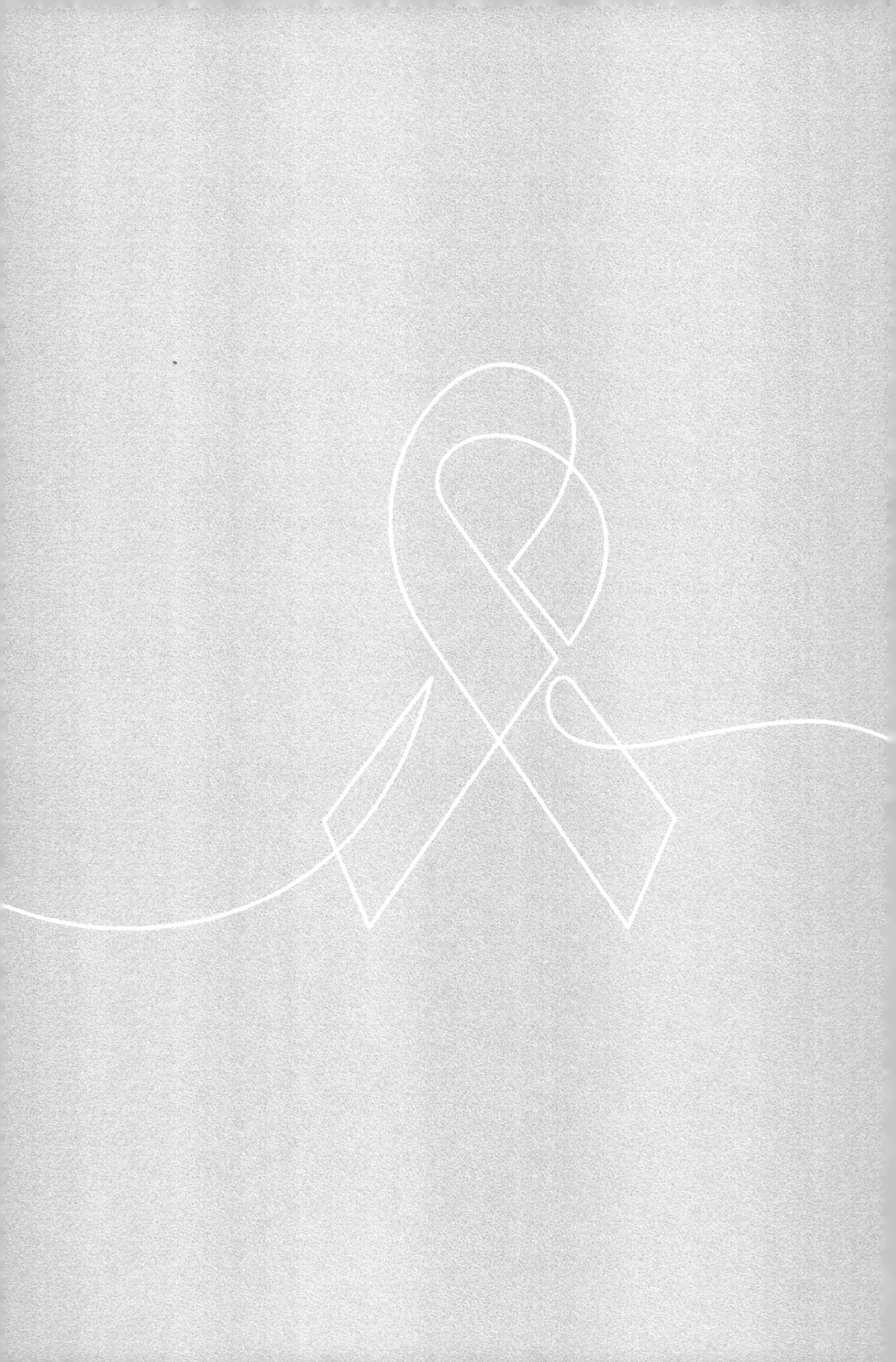

TerriLyn

"Many people will walk in and out of your life, but only true friends leave footprints in your heart."

—Eleanor Roosevelt

TerriLyn died today.

I told Michael, "The way I am feeling is not sustainable, my friend is gone."

I'm exhausted, sad, and I feel overwhelming defeat. My brain and my heart are disconnected. Cerebrally, I knew her body was breaking down. – *Failing,* a word I don't use often nor like, but regardless of my opinion, that is exactly what was happening, her body was shutting down.

TerriLyn and I still had plans for the future. We were co-survivors and our plans included bringing light to others; and sharing the abundance of life even when we were faced with adversity.

I suddenly found myself shutting down too. I had only enough in me for my family and some for TerriLyn's. I spent daylight hours with mine and evening hours with hers.

The last time we spoke outside of the hospital, was in a restaurant. This is a fitting setting for our meeting. She was greeted warmly by our waitress as they discussed TerriLyn's favorite items on the menu. They shared a communication encrypted with *foodisms* I was unfamiliar with.

"Would you like that sauce…" The waitress didn't finish her question.

"I would. Is it sweet like the…"

"As always, we'll serve it warm—just as you like it – with a side order of…"

"Perfect!" TerriLyn did not need to finish her order.

I was at a loss and eager to see just what was going to be delivered! I've always admired these connections TerriLyn had with people.

If the rest of the world operated in a *Six Degrees of Separation*, then TerriLyn operated in a world separated by only *four degrees*.

But now she is gone and the feeling I am experiencing is unexpected emptiness. I thought I was prepared.

My typical *M.O.* is to put my feelings into something tangible, into action, rather than stewing.

So, I move my body. I practice yoga to literally move the energy of emotion around inside. I hike so that I can expel breath from my body. I laugh during funny movies so that I can feel *lightness* again.

Yet, I find myself returning back to dread and the realization that she was gone.

"Ugh!" I was frustrated.

I scheduled myself for some body work with my friend, Rose. She had the opportunity to work on TerriLyn's body while exchanging stories that bonded them to certain common life experiences. Once again, the heart strings of TerriLyn had hooked another soul. Rose, lovingly, made herself available for me.

I turn to the lessons that I have learned.

TerriLyn and I had planned to write it this book together. We would meet weekly at a coffee shop to swap stories and devise a lesson plan, so to speak. We would make notes about what helped us to face the challenges that coincide with surgeries, chemotherapy, radiation, and publicly venturing out into the world completely bald. We shared experiences that both differed and those that were similar, but we always ended in the same place.

The bottom line to this cancer adventure of ours, and perhaps for others too, relied on one very important trait—humor.

As food establishments consistently provided us with the perfect venue for creativity and the exchange of personal experiences, we shared what we knew to be true to our own sustainability, laughter. Somehow, instinctively, we each knew that we would drown in our own sorrow if we could not locate this place in our heart.

TerriLyn's sister, Julie, spoke at her funeral. Once again, a wave of laughter bathed the room of five hundred plus of friends and family members as Julie revealed childhood events consistent with the person that I had come to know as my friend. She told a story about TL's (one of her nicknames) life in Boston where she worked as a barista at a coffee cart.

She had traveled to Boston for a bicycle seeking adventure. She was indoctrinated to her new home and place of adventure when her bike was stolen shortly after her arrival. Her parents, wanting to support their daughter, bought her a car. A car in Boston can be a great thing, until you need to park it. TerriLyn received so many parking tickets in one year that she donned all of them for a Halloween costume and arrived at her party as one big parking ticket.

And then the car was stolen!

Her Boston adventure was well on its way when she met two regular coffee customers who took TerriLyn under their wing, showing her some of the marvels of the east coast thereby counteracting some of the Boston drama. They opened up their Maine cabin to TL, giving her the opportunity to work as a ski instructor for one winter.

Their friendship grew stronger and, once again, TerriLyn had hooked her heart strings into the hearts of this couple. As Julie relayed this Boston adventure, it was apparent this couple had not known the impact that they had made on TerriLyn's life.

TerriLyn's older brother, Gary, spoke about the family humor gene living large in his own childhood memory. Recalling big brother stroller rides with TL as the baby passenger, afternoon football practices with their eldest brother, both boys completely geared-up and TL only in her PJs.

Sitting in the audience amongst my friends, my emotions waxing and waning, riding my roller coaster of feelings so abundantly, I actually became concerned that I would get to a place where I would be feeling too much.

Gary closed his childhood tormenting stories of his younger sister with an endearing event that occurred to him only recently. Gary lives and works in his hometown of Seattle, Washington. He relayed to all of the moist eyes in the room his encounter with a man who lives with a disability so severe that it impedes his walking journey to work each morning; and yet, this man chooses to make that journey each day. Gary thought he was younger than he was, but it was difficult to tell as his physical stature was so badly bent, and his eyes held years of living in a body that half-worked. Being rainy Seattle, Gary often stopped when he saw this man and offered him a car ride to work.

Occasionally he took Gary up on his offer.

On one of these rainy days when Gary and this man shared a fairly silent ride, TL's brother initiated the conversation with morning small talk, commenting on the weather, asking questions about this man's job, etc. When Gary forgot this man's name, he offered his own name first before asking again.

The man said his name was Sam and then paused when he heard Gary's last name.

Sam asked, "Are you related to TerriLyn Folkman?"

Somewhat surprised, Gary said, "Yes. She's my sister."

Sam adjusted in his seat and then looked at Gary. "She was the only one who treated me with any kindness and respect when we were in high school together."

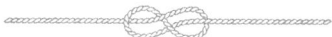

In my attempt to make sense of this particular ending of my meetings with TerriLyn, I turn to my teachings of yoga. I cannot honestly say that my relationship with her has ended.

The Yoga Nataraj is a statue that depicts Shiva, a Hindu deity, as a dancer with four arms. The dance refers to the constant cycle of birth and death, sustaining and evolving, which happens with all things. We set ourselves up for disappointment if we attach ourselves to any part of this cycle and lose sight that everything is in a constant flux of change.

It's like trying to enjoy the scenic view while riding the Scrambler, that diabolic amusement park ride designed to spin you mercilessly in circles, eventually scrambling your brain, or making you puke, or both. The Nataraj suggests that everything is turning, changing as we speak. Just as things are dying, something else is being born, opening up the heart to reveal something new—*Revealing Grace.*

While keeping TerriLyn company in her hospital room, my job was to provide her comfort, so I rubbed her feet with essential oils and played soft music. It was in these final days of her life, while hooked up to tubes and wires and appearing jaundice, that I witnessed an army of people.

TerriLyn's community entered her room with the intent of comforting her. But in reality, it was TerriLyn who ended up comforting them, revealed HER grace, and provided the strength that this community of people needed.

As I write, I sit at my computer and watch the screen as the words appear. There is not a day that goes by that I don't think of my friend, TerriLyn. She is sitting beside me and oftentimes within me. She helped build our QLC community and is mentioned (as are the others who are no longer with us) each year as we honor one another during our annual Grand American high tea visits.

As Rose often reminded me, "Energy never dies—it just changes form."

Shaker song, eighteenth century *Oremus Hymnal*

'Tis the gift to be simple,

'tis the gift to be free,

'tis the gift to come down,

where we ought to be,

and when we find ourselves in the place just right,

'twill be in the valley of love and delight.

When true simplicity is gained,

to bow and to bend we shan't be ashamed,

to turn, turn, will be our delight,

till by turning, turning we come round right.

Blessing

And through and over everything, a sense of glad awakening.
—Edna St. Vincent Millay

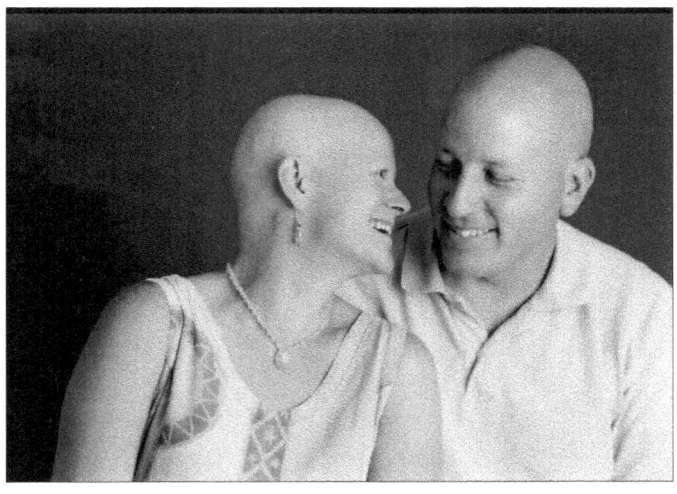

In trying to make sense of serious illnesses, you can make yourself crazy. Was there a reason for breast cancer to enter my life when it did?

The discovery of my tumor occurred during the time around my daughter's birthday in March 2005, and treatment ended during the time around my son's birthday in November of the same year; nine months, the gestational period for new life.

My life has changed considerably since that critical day in March. By the time Thanksgiving fell upon us, I no longer took my days for granted. I no longer played the comparison game. What a waste of time that was!

I listened better. I reached out farther. I held closer.

Colors became more glorious, the mountains more spectacular. Our time together much more valuable than a roundtrip ticket to Europe.

What if the reason for the cancer diagnosis was to help me see and pursue these things? My world is broader, my vision longer, my desires more intense, my beliefs stronger.

"Was cancer a blessing?"

Whew! I had to breathe through that one.

I often commented to Michael that I wasn't sure if I could do the whole treatment thing over again. It was hard. I had to dig down deep to keep my wits about me.

I don't believe that cancer itself was a blessing, but the change that impacted my life, well, there is no doubt in my mind, *that was a blessing.*

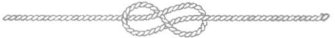

> "Too often we underestimate the power of a touch,
> a smile, a kind word, a listening ear, an honest
> compliment, or the smallest act of caring,
> all of which have the potential to turn a life around."
>
> —Leo Buscaglia

ABOUT THE AUTHOR

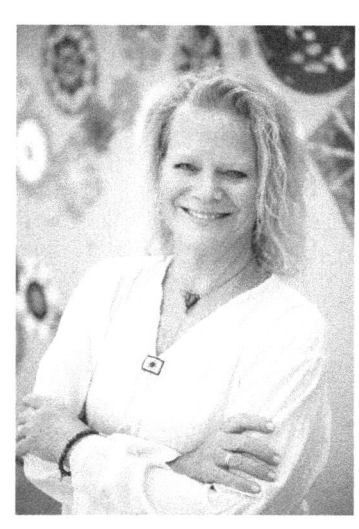

In April 2005, *The Salt Lake Tribune* featured Amy Conn on the front page of the Sport's section, Running through Adversity. "Amy Conn will run the Salt Lake City Marathon four days before undergoing chemotherapy and one month following a lumpectomy."

Amy retired from teaching public-school after thirty-four years where she was a Reading Specialist. She has degrees in Special Education for Deaf and Hard of Hearing, as well as Exercise and Sports Science.

She works with the University of Utah as a yoga instructor at their Burn Unit Camps, with Survivor Wellness for cancer survivors, and Mindfulness Based Stress Reduction for Teenagers (MBSR-T). Lastly, Amy is a Master Level Intuitive Reiki practitioner.

This 2nd edition publication covers her volunteer advocacy in Washington, D.C., where she was a lobbyist for rights on behalf of cancer survivors to raise funds for American Cancer Society.

Amy currently runs yearly writing and yoga retreats in addition to writing a weekly newsletter/blog spanning various topics of Wellness at **amyconnyoga.com/blog**.

She currently lives in Salt Lake City, Utah with her Firefighter husband, Michael. Her two children are chasing their dreams as a pilot in Anchorage, Alaska and as an Equine Therapist in Minnesota.

Amy Conn
amyconnyoga@gmail.com
amyconnyoga.com

Acknowledgments

I offer my gratitude to these beautiful writers and book editors: Dawn Brockett, Lavina Anderson, Brent Corcoran, Lisa Groen, Rolf & Marian Gates and KK Baker; you guided me through significant periods of my life and this story.

I give thanks to my doctors who offer their expertise, wisdom, kindness and sensitivity: Drs. Anna Beck, Cynthia Cannon, Regina Rosenthal, Brett Parkinson, Nitin Chandramouli, and Leslie Peterson; thank you for treating me like a person first and your patient second.

I extend endless amounts of gratitude (along with patience) to my technical support team: Russ and Liz Martin, James Burris, Mike Bates, David Miller, Cree Putney & Joannie Packard; ALL of you deserve a trip to Napa Valley (on me!)

To those who have helped me financially and legally: Chris Putney, Clovis and Sue Putney, and Adam Grundvig; I don't know how anyone can complete this dream without family and friends.

I honor my guides of heart, mind and spirit: Carolyn Paquette, KK Baker, Barbara Ljord, TerriLyn Grundvig, Julia Kuznetsov, Pam Humen, Florence "Aunty" Petris, and Caitlyn Putney; friends and family from long ago and today—you've given me insight and courage to keep writing and to keep feeling.

To friends who fed our family with food and much, much more: Julia Hamilton, Mark & Laurie Bolt, Kent & Jean Smith, Chris & Sarah Macdonald, Jesse & Joie Nutting, Terry Crandall, Marion "Merb" Jones, Thomas Johnson & Tina Bond, Dennis & Maggie Tesch, Nick and Jolie Strohmeyer, Alex & Amy Bocock, Michelle Bradshaw, Mark & Jean Resetarits, Annabel Sheinberg and running mate Paige Beals!

Acknowledgments

To all who lent their talents and mentoring skills toward crafting this book: Richard Paul Evans, Celeste Edmunds, Debbie Rasmussen, Scott Moore, Kim Autrey, and Francine Platt.

Finally, to my family: Michael, Benjamin and Abigail Conn. You are the bravest people I know. I'm honored to be your wife and mother. To Clovis & Sue Putney, Claude & Connie Conn, Lee & Debbie Cox, Cree Putney & Terrie Stoner, Jimmie & Cheryl Mayhand, Chris & Mary Ann Putney, Pam & Bob Humen, Douglas & Alisa Hubbard, David & Jackie Miller and all the nieces and nephews – I love you all!

To view the photos in color, including more photos than were included in this book, please visit **amyconnyoga.com/book**

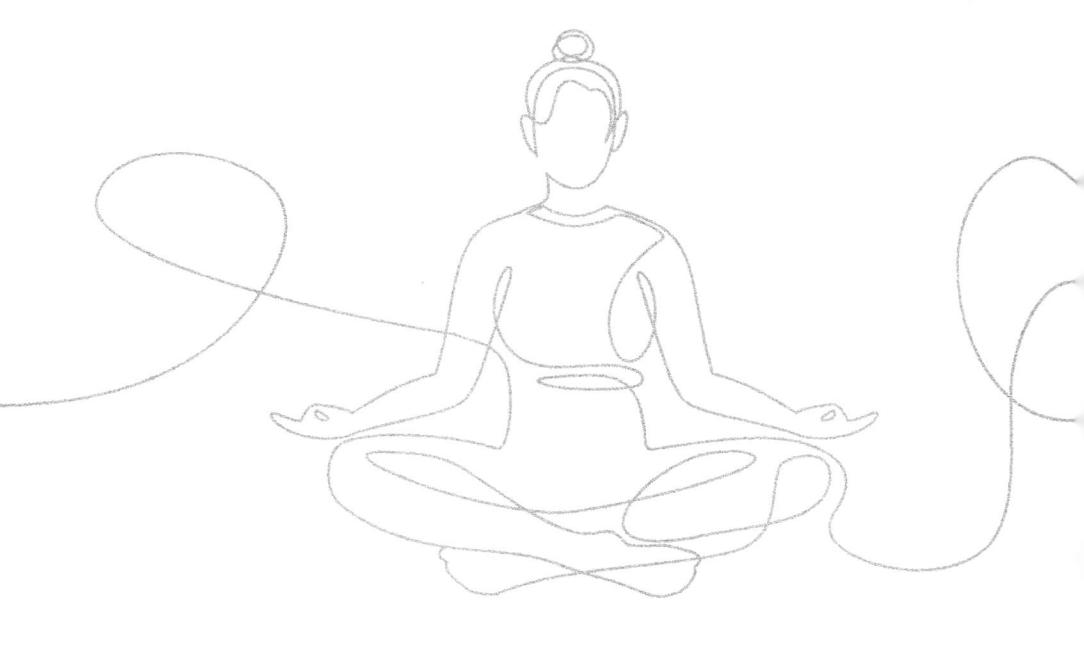